VEGETARIAN

INSTANT POT COOKBOOK 2019

Instant Pot Vegetarian for Beginners with 101 Easy, Delicious Vegetarian Recipes to Live A Healthy Lifestyle

By Mohali Smith

Table of Content

Scrumptious Dessert Recipes

INTRODUCTION

In creating this cookbook of vegetarian recipes for the Instant Pot, we took a large amount of time to consider our audience. Who is most likely to be interested in this book and want to cook from it? There are many reasons that someone might choose a vegetarian diet. With the rise in health issues, increasing interest in environmental sustainability, concerns for animal welfare, and growing prices of meat, the movement for a more plant-based diet is gaining in popularity.

Whether you are a new vegetarian who is wondering where to begin or someone seasoned to this way of eating, this comprehensive cookbook will give you fresh ideas that will keep you fed for years down the road. Forget trying to modify omnivorous recipes with ultra-processed alternative meat products; the recipes in this cookbook were tailored for you. With recipes centered around whole food plant-based staples, such as legumes, whole grains, fruits, vegetables, nuts, and seeds, this book can help whether your main goal is to completely omit meat or simply to incorporate more plants. You'll learn the basics of constructing a fortifying vegetarian meal, as well as techniques to build flavor. This wide-ranging collection of 101 recipes includes everything from soups and salads, to grain and legume combinations, as well as egg dishes for those who choose to eat eggs. The recipes for beverages, snacks, and desserts provide the finishing touches to your meal. This book has you covered whether you are craving items like comforting and familiar vegetable noodle soup, or something more exotic, such as Swedish glogg.

Ready to make a hearty vegetarian dinner the centerpiece of your table? Head over to the section on "Flavorful Rice, Beans, and Lentils," where you can choose from a variety of satisfying curries and grain-based dishes. How does coconut red lentil curry sound? What about a creamy mushroom alfredo rice? You'll have a veritable feast on your hands when you pair these entrees with dishes in the other chapters that work well as starters and sides, but can also stand-alone if you are looking for a lighter meal. Check out the "Nutritional Vegetables" section for dishes like nutty Brussels sprouts salad and spicy cauliflower that will enliven any meal. We've included the number of servings as well as the preparation and cook time, so you'll be able to plan the right amount of food and time things so the meal is ready when you need it.

Because we wanted to make this book a complete vegetarian guide for Instant Pot users, we didn't leave out the simple recipes like tomato soup, simple broccoli, and spiced nuts. Good home cooks rely on the basics like these as cornerstone recipes to make great meals and snacks. Many people are busy and cannot create a four-course dinner from scratch every night but relying on a few basic principles will help you to get easy and healthful meals on the table fast. If eggs fit your way of eating, don't miss out on the "Innovative Eggs" recipe section for versatile dishes that include this high-quality protein. Eggs make a great base for a simple breakfast, lunch, or dinner.

Whether you are new to plant-based cooking or well-practiced, we hope that you find cooking from this book to be an enjoyable experience. If we've inspired you to try an ingredient that is new to you or to cook with familiar ingredients in new ways, and if the book has helped to develop your interest in vegetarian cooking and you are having fun, we have accomplished our goal. Wondering where to get started on this culinary adventure? How about taking your taste buds on a trip across the globe with some comforting manchow soup? If that doesn't suit your fancy, why not try quinoa pilaf, a change up on the classic rice-based dish that increases the protein and iron content. This book is packed with easy to follow recipes that will make you curious about food, and possibly inspire trips to the farmer's market and ethnic grocery stores in your area, in search of different types of greens, spices, beans, and grains. You won't miss the meat in these dishes that will have you exploring novel ways to build delicious flavors.

It can be tough to please all of the palates in a crowd, but our recipe testers have worked hard to create dishes that have universal appeal. To get you started, keep reading for suggestions of ingredients to keep on hand to put together a well-stocked vegetarian pantry and make the most of your Instant Pot. Before long, you'll be a pro at putting together beautiful vegetarian meals that are worthy of top notch restaurants. Are you ready? Then let's get started!

SECTION ONE:
VEGETARIAN BASICS

Essential Ingredients

Don't turn on your Instant Pot just yet! Before you get cooking, it is important to ensure that your refrigerator and pantry are stocked with the foods and ingredients that you need to put together the recipes in this cookbook. Wouldn't it be inconvenient to get halfway through a recipe only to realize you need an onion or a certain spice and have to run to the store? By planning ahead, you can save yourself time in constructing meals. Here are some items that we recommend having on hand:

- Fruits and vegetables (your favorites and some new ones)
- Grains such as rice, quinoa, and pasta
- Legumes (including products made from soy such as tofu and tempeh)
- Dairy foods or calcium-fortified dairy alternatives (milks, cheeses, and yogurt)
- Eggs
- Nuts and seeds
- Mushrooms (both fresh and dried)
- Assorted oils and vinegars
- Vegetable broth or homemade vegetable stock
- Soy sauce or liquid aminos
- Tomato puree
- Citrus juice
- Spices and fresh herbs

Ensuring Nutritional Needs are Being Met on a Vegetarian Diet

A well-planned vegetarian diet that includes dairy products and eggs can easily meet a person's needs for all essential nutrients. It is important that the diet be well constructed because a diet filled with mostly nutrient-poor foods, whether vegetarian or not, can result in deficiencies. A vegetarian diet pattern is currently one of the three diet patterns suggested in the Dietary Guidelines for Americans that is linked to long-term health. There are no essential nutrients in meat, poultry, and fish that cannot be covered by a balanced diet of dairy, eggs, and plant foods.

For those who have limited lactose tolerance, dairy allergy, or who choose to eschew dairy for other reasons, choosing calcium-fortified dairy alternatives can ensure adequate intake of this bone-building mineral. Another issue to be aware of is that the non-heme iron in plant foods is not as readily absorbed as the heme iron in animal foods, so vegetarians have nearly twice the Recommended Dietary Allowance (RDA) for iron compared to omnivores. One way to help increase the absorption of non-heme iron is to include foods rich in vitamin C in your meals along with the foods containing iron. Flavoring iron-rich legumes and grains with citrus juices is one easy way to accomplish this.

As far as other micronutrients are concerned, meats are a rich source of many of the B vitamins, but so are many grains. Grains (and all other plant foods) are naturally lacking in vitamin B12, so it is important to choose foods that are fortified with this nutrient (such as nutritional yeast and some breakfast cereals), and consider taking a supplement if you do not eat animal products. Though the essential omega-3 ALA is plentiful in certain plant foods such as walnuts and flax seeds, EPA and DHA may be lacking in vegetarian diets. Choose products such as eggs from chickens fed omega-3 rich chicken feed, DHA-fortified tofu, or an algal oil supplement if you would like to increase intake of DHA on a vegetarian diet.

Because vitamin C, beta-carotene, folate, and fiber tend to be plentiful in fruits and vegetables these dietary components tend to be abundant in the vegetarian diet. Non-essential phytonutrients that are linked to long-term health are also plentiful in the fruits and vegetables included in the vegetarian diet. Though some vitamin D may be found in dairy foods as well as mushrooms treated with UV-light, there is a paucity of natural food sources of vitamin D (for vegetarians and omnivores alike), so ask your doctor about supplementing with this nutrient if you have low blood levels.

In order to be a healthy vegetarian, all of the above factors should be taken into account to get a balanced diet comprising different foods. An example menu is given below. One advantage of plant-based proteins is that they tend to be much lower in saturated fat than animal-based proteins. Plant proteins, unlike animal proteins, contain fiber that can benefit digestion and the gut microbiome as well.

There is a potentially higher risk of nutrient deficiencies with more restrictive vegan diets, as opposed to lacto-ovo vegetarian diets (diet definitions can be found below). Aside from ensuring adequate vitamin B12 intake, it is particularly important for vegans to pay attention to the nutrients which are key to bone health, since vegans are at a higher risk of low bone mineral density and fractures. Some key bone-supporting nutrients include calcium, vitamin D, vitamin K2, magnesium, and phosphorus. These issues can be overcome; being well-informed about nutrition is the key point in remaining healthy.

Sample Meal Plan for Vegetarians

Breakfast

- Dairy product or calcium-fortified milk alternative
- Cereals or whole grains
- Protein from eggs or legumes
- Fruits

Lunch

- Dairy product or calcium-fortified milk alternative
- Whole grain or enriched/fortified refined grain
- Protein from legumes
- Salad packed with leafy greens, an assortment of other vegetables and/or fruits, and a healthy fat (nuts or seeds)

Dinner

- Dairy product or calcium-fortified milk alternative
- Whole grain or enriched/fortified refined grain
- Protein from legumes
- Vegetable side dish(es) served with healthy fat (nuts or seeds)

Steps to Achieve Recommended Dietary Allowance:

- Consume 3 servings of milk or a calcium-fortified milk alternative daily
- Use snacks to fill in the gaps in your diet (e.g., have fruits for snacks if you are not consuming enough fruit)
- If you do not eat eggs, aim to get several servings of soy foods per day to get adequate choline. One easy way to do this is to choose a soy-based calcium-fortified milk alternative.

- Don't forget the healthy fats from nuts and seeds like almonds and pumpkin seeds.
- It is important for vegetarians to consume a variety of grains and legumes each day to help ensure that they are getting adequate amounts of all of the essential amino acids in the diet.

Types of Vegetarian Diets

Vegetarianism has a long history that continues to our present day. Over 3% of Americans consider themselves vegans or vegetarians, including a particularly large population of young adult females. Not everyone who adopts this diet does so solely for wellness. Some, such as the Seventh-day Adventists, choose vegetarianism for religious and/or cultural reasons. Others adopt this way of eating because they are interested in environmentally sustainable dietary patterns and reducing their carbon footprint. Some have ethical concerns over the treatment of animals and animal welfare. Many who adopt the vegetarian way of eating do so for multiple reasons.

The vegetarian diet is not a singular diet. There are actually various types of vegetarian diets and the degree of restriction varies from one type to the other. Here are some of the most common types of vegetarian diets that you should know about:

Lacto-ovo Vegetarian: This is the most widely-adopted type of vegetarian diet. It excludes consuming meat, poultry, and fish, but allows consuming other animal-derived products such as eggs, dairy products, and honey.

Lacto Vegetarian: A diet which excludes all animal-derived products except dairy is called a lacto vegetarian diet.

Ovo Vegetarian: A diet which excludes all animal-derived products except eggs is called an ovo vegetarian diet.

Pescatarian Diet: A diet which excludes meat and poultry but not fish is called a pescatarian diet. Pescatarians generally consume dairy products, eggs, and honey as well.

Vegan Diet: A diet which excludes all kinds of animal and animal-derived products is called a vegan diet. Vegans typically aim to eliminate as many animal-derived products from their lives as possible, including non-edible products such as leather shoes and belts.

Plant-based Diet: The term "plant-based diet" means different things to different people, so be sure to ask for greater clarification if someone identifies this as their way of eating. In some cases the person may mean a vegetarian diet, while in others, they simply mean they eat mostly plant foods.

SECTION TWO: INSTANT POT BASICS

What is the Instant Pot?

With the advancement of technology in almost every field, culinary and kitchen-related appliances have also been gaining ground from time to time. One such innovative appliance is the Instant Pot. It is a high-tech conglomeration of several of your favorite kitchen appliances combined into one. Its versatility and ability to turn low-cost ingredients (such as dried beans and whole grains) into fast, wholesome meals makes it an appealing choice to add to your kitchen.

Cooking Functions of the Instant Pot

In a world where ultra-processed foods and restaurant meals are easier than cooking yourself some delicious food, the Instant Pot is going to make life easier with surprisingly quick and healthy cooked food. With so many public health campaigns being focused on health issues and consuming a healthy diet, the Instant Pot just might be the solution the harried person was looking for. Though this culinary wonder may vary slightly by model, most Instant Pots offer the following cooking functions:

- Pressure cooker
- Slow cooker

- Rice cooker

- Steamer

- Sauté

- Yogurt maker

- Food warmer

This single pot appliance will replace multiple larger appliances, a blessing for those with a small kitchen. With the pressure cooker function, you'll be able to shave hours off of the cooking time for time-consuming ingredients such as dried beans. You'll appreciate your new ability to get nutrient-rich food on the table fast, whether you mostly cook for yourself or are feeding a crowd.

The Benefits of Instant Pot

Being a 7-in-1 appliance is not the only benefit of the revolutionary Instant Pot. There are a number of reasons why you should switch to pressure cooking with this appliance:

It's Time Efficient- If you are a busy worker (and who isn't nowadays) then your time is most likely pretty limited. The instant pot can provide you with the chance to start home cooking again because it actually cooks the meals 70 percent faster than other appliances.

It Saves Money- Another benefit of the Instant Pot is the fact that it saves energy. Cooking 70 percent faster means using 70 percent less energy than other appliances, which cuts your electric bill significantly. Another way in which the Instant Pot can save you money is that it turns even the least expensive ingredients, like dried beans and grains, into restaurant-worthy incredible dishes.

Even Cooking- Thanks to the pressure flow inside the pot, the meals are cooked evenly, with no undercooked parts or edges that are burnt.

Greater Digestibility- Pressure cooking means cooking at a temperature that is higher than the point of boiling water. This method of cooking is great for those who get some GI upset after consuming beans; the compounds in the beans which cause the disturbance are reduced, resulting in more comfortable digestion.

It is Convenient- Cooking has really never been easier. You can simply dump your ingredients in the pot, close the lid, set the cooking mode and time, and you will get delicious results in minutes.

So, if your busy routine is not allowing you in having a healthy and balanced diet, an Instant Pot is going to provide you with nutrient-rich meals in a short amount of time. This could be the turning point in helping you achieve a health-promoting life style. Is it any surprise that the Instant Pot has received amazing reviews from users on Amazon? Cooking has been revolutionized with its advent and the world is unable to resist it.

Instant Pot Cooking Chart for Common Vegetables

The following cooking chart has been adapted from the Instant Pot website. This is for a small or medium amount of vegetables; be sure to add more water and increase the cooking time if you wish to cook larger portions.

Vegetable	Fresh, Cooking Time (in Minutes)	Frozen, Cooking Time (in Minutes)
Asparagus, whole or cut	1 – 2	2 – 3
Broccoli, flowerets	2 – 3	3 – 4
Brussel sprouts, whole	3 – 4	4 – 5
Carrots, whole or chunked	2 – 3	3 – 4
Cauliflower flowerets	2 – 3	3 – 4
Corn, kernels	1 – 2	2 – 3
Eggplant, slices or chunks	2 – 3	3 – 4
Green beans, whole	2 – 3	3 – 4
Greens (beet greens, collards, kale, spinach, swiss chard, turnip greens), chopped	3 – 6	4 – 7
Mixed vegetables	2 – 3	3 – 4
Onions, sliced	2 – 3	3 – 4
Peas, green	1 – 2	2 – 3
Potatoes, in cubes	7 – 9	9 – 11
Squash, butternut, slices or chunks	8 – 10	10 – 12
Sweet potato, in cubes	7 – 9	9 – 11
Tomatoes, in quarters	2 – 3	4 – 5
Tomatoes, whole	3 – 5	5 – 7
Zucchini, slices or chunks	2 – 3	3 – 4

Cleaning and Maintenance Tips for the Instant Pot

➤ Follow the recommendations in the user's manual of your Instant Pot model for specific tips for cleaning and maintenance.

➤ Always unplug your Instant Pot and make sure it is cool before cleaning.

➤ The cooking pot, steam rack, and lid are dishwasher safe. If your inner pot has hard water stains, try removing them with a damp sponge that was soaked in vinegar.

➤ Do not use steel wool to clean your Instant Pot. It may damage the surfaces.

➤ The stainless steel exterior should be wiped clean with a damp cloth, not put in the dishwasher. The exterior is fingerprint resistant, to maintain its appearance.

➤ For proper maintenance of your Instant Pot, never fill it past the interior 2/3 mark.

➤ Make sure to add the amount of liquid called for in the recipe before starting the pressure cooking function.

➤ Always note the total cooking time.

➤ Take care of your Instant Pot, and it will take care of your cooking needs for years to come!

NUTRITIONAL VEGETABLES RECIPES

1.Brussels Sprout Salad

Yield: 4 Servings, Prep Time: 10 Minutes, Cook Time: 5 Minutes

Ingredients

- 1 pound Brussels sprouts, trimmed and halved
- ¼ cup cashew nuts, chopped
- ½ tablespoon unsalted butter, melted
- ¼ cup almonds, chopped
- 1 cup pomegranate seeds
- 1 cup water
- Salt and black pepper, to taste

Directions

1. Place the steamer trivet in the bottom of Instant Pot and add water.
2. Season the Brussels sprout with salt and pepper, then put them on the trivet.
3. Set the Instant Pot to "Manual" at high pressure for 4 minutes.
4. Release the pressure naturally and open the lid.
5. Top with melted butter, almonds, cashew nuts and pomegranate seeds.
6. Mix well and serve.

Nutritional Information per Serving:

Calories: 170; Total Fat: 8.8g; Carbs: 20.4g; Sugars: 6.1g; Protein: 6.7g; Cholesterol: 4mg; Sodium: 42mg

2.Whole Garlic Roast

Yield: 4 Servings, Prep Time: 2 Minutes, Cook Time: 9 Minutes

Ingredients

- 4 large garlic bulbs
- 2 tablespoons herbed butter
- 1 cup water
- Salt and black pepper, to taste

Directions

1. Place the steamer trivet in the bottom of Instant Pot and add water.
2. Season the garlic bulbs with salt and pepper.
3. Put the seasoned garlic bulbs on the trivet.
4. Set the Instant Pot to "Manual" at high pressure for 6 minutes.
5. Release the pressure naturally and remove the trivet.
6. Put the herbed butter and garlic bulbs and select "Sauté".
7. Sauté for 3 minutes and dish out.

Nutritional Information per Serving:

Calories: 66; Total Fat: 5.8g; Carbs: 3g; Sugars: 0g; Protein: 0.1g; Cholesterol: 15mg; Sodium: 43mg

3.Tangy Lemon Potatoes

Yield: 6 Servings, Prep Time: 3 Minutes, Cook Time: 12 Minutes

Ingredients

- 10 medium potatoes, scrubbed and cubed
- 4 tablespoons fresh lemon juice
- 2 tablespoons olive oil
- 4 tablespoons fresh rosemary, chopped
- 2 cups vegetable broth
- Salt and black pepper, to taste

Directions:

1. Put the olive oil and potatoes in the Instant Pot and select "Sauté".
2. Sauté for 4 minutes and add the rosemary, salt and black pepper.
3. Sauté for 2 minutes and stir in the lemon juice and broth.
4. Set the Instant Pot to "Manual" at high pressure for 6 minutes.
5. Release the pressure naturally and serve warm.

Nutritional Information per Serving:

Calories: 307; Total Fat: 5.9g; Carbs: 57.7g; Sugars: 4.5g; Protein: 7.8g; Cholesterol: 0mg; Sodium: 279mg

4.Caramelised Onions

Yield: 2 Servings, Prep Time: 3 Minutes, Cook Time: 9 Minutes

Ingredients

- 3 large onion bulbs
- 1 cup water
- 1 tablespoon butter
- Salt and black pepper, to taste

Directions:

1. Place the steamer trivet in the bottom of Instant Pot and add water.
2. Season the onion bulbs with salt and pepper.
3. Put the seasoned onion bulbs on the trivet.
4. Set the Instant Pot to "Manual" at high pressure for 6 minutes.
5. Release the pressure naturally and remove the trivet.
6. Put the butter and garlic bulbs and select "Sauté".
7. Sauté for 3 minutes and dish out.

Nutritional Information per Serving:

Calories: 63; Total Fat: 5.8g; Carbs: 2.8g; Sugars: 0.9g; Protein: 0.8g; Cholesterol: 0mg; Sodium: 50mg

5.Tomato Sauce Spinach

Yield: 4 Servings, Prep Time: 5 Minutes, Cook Time: 13 Minutes

Ingredients

- 1 tablespoon olive oil
- 1 small onion, chopped
- 1 teaspoon garlic, minced
- ½ teaspoon red pepper flakes, crushed
- 5 cups fresh spinach, chopped
- ½ cup tomatoes, chopped
- ¼ cup homemade tomato puree
- ¼ cup white wine
- ½ cup vegetable broth

Directions:

1. Put the olive oil and onions in the Instant Pot and select "Sauté".
2. Sauté for 4 minutes and add garlic, spinach and red pepper flakes.
3. Sauté for 3 minutes and stir in the remaining ingredients.
4. Set the Instant Pot to "Manual" at high pressure for 6 minutes.
5. Release the pressure quickly and serve warm.

Nutritional Information per Serving:

Calories: 72; Total Fat: 3.9g; Carbs: 5.5g; Sugars: 2.2g; Protein: 2.3g; Cholesterol: 0mg; Sodium: 130mg

6.Glazed Carrots

Yield: 3 Servings, Prep Time: 5 Minutes, Cook Time: 5 Minutes

Ingredients

- 1 pound carrots, peeled and sliced diagonally
- ½ cup water
- 1 tablespoon honey
- ¼ cup golden raisins
- 1 tablespoon unsalted butter, melted
- ½ teaspoon red pepper flakes, crushed
- Pinch of salt

Directions

1. Put the carrots, water and raisins in the Instant Pot.
2. Set the Instant Pot to "Manual" at low pressure for 5 minutes.
3. Release the pressure naturally and transfer he carrots into a bowl.
4. Stir in the remaining ingredients and mix well to serve.

Nutritional Information per Serving:

Calories: 154; Total Fat: 4g; Carbs: 30.4g; Sugars: 20.4g; Protein: 1.7g; Cholesterol: 10mg; Sodium: 134mg

7.Rosemary Baby Potatoes

Yield: 7 Servings, Prep Time: 5 Minutes, Cook Time: 15 Minutes

Ingredients

- 20 baby potatoes
- 2 cups water
- 1 cup fresh rosemary
- 4tablespoons herb butter

Directions:

1. Place the steamer trivet in the bottom of Instant Pot and add water.
2. Put the baby potatoes and rosemary on the trivet.
3. Set the Instant Pot to "Manual" at high pressure for 10 minutes.
4. Release the pressure naturally and remove the trivet.
5. Put the herbed butter and baby potatoes and select "Sauté".
6. Sauté for 5 minutes and dish out.

Nutritional Information per Serving:

Calories: 108; Total Fat: 1.7g; Carbs: 22.1g; Sugars: 0g; Protein: 3.6g; Cholesterol: 1mg; Sodium: 77mg

8.Chili Polenta

Yield: 6 Servings, Prep Time: 5 Minutes, Cook Time: 10 Minutes

Ingredients

- 3 cups coarse polenta
- 10 cups water
- 3 teaspoons salt
- 3tablespoons red paprika flakes

Directions:

1. Put the water, salt, red paprika flakes and polenta flour in the Instant Pot.
2. Set the Instant Pot to "Manual" at high pressure for 9 minutes.
3. Release the pressure naturally and dish out.

Nutritional Information per Serving:

Calories: 310; Total Fat: 9.7g; Carbs: 66.8g; Sugars: 0.8g; Protein: 5.8g; Cholesterol: 0mg; Sodium: 1178mg

9.Steamed Cabbage Sheets

Yield: 4 Servings, Prep Time: 6 Minutes, Cook Time: 9 Minutes

Ingredients

- 12 sheets of fresh cabbage
- 3 teaspoons fresh basil
- 3 teaspoons olive oil
- 2 cups water
- Salt and pepper

Directions:

1. Place the steamer trivet in the bottom of Instant Pot and add water.
2. Put the cabbage sheets and basil on the trivet.
3. Set the Instant Pot to "Manual" at high pressure for 6 minutes.
4. Release the pressure naturally and remove the trivet.
5. Put the olive oil, cabbage sheets, salt and black pepper and select "Sauté".
6. Sauté for 3 minutes and dish out.

Nutritional Information per Serving:

Calories: 55; Total Fat: 3.6g; Carbs: 5.8g; Sugars: 3.2g; Protein: 1.3g; Cholesterol: 0mg; Sodium: 21mg

10.Instant Pot Corn Kernels

Yield: 4 Servings, Prep Time: 5 Minutes, Cook Time: 8 Minutes

Ingredients

- 1½ cups corn kernels
- 2 cups water
- 1 tablespoons lemon juice
- 2 tablespoons butter
- 1 teaspoon red pepper powder
- Salt and black pepper, to taste

Directions:

1. Season the corn kernels with red pepper powder, salt and black pepper
2. Place the steamer trivet in the bottom of Instant Pot and add water.
3. Put the seasoned corn kernels on the trivet.
4. Set the Instant Pot to "Manual" at high pressure for 5 minutes.
5. Release the pressure naturally and remove the trivet.
6. Put the butter and corn kernels and select "Sauté".
7. Sauté for 3 minutes and stir in the lemon juice.

Nutritional Information per Serving:

Calories: 188; Total Fat: 6.7g; Carbs: 32.2g; Sugars: 5.6g; Protein: 5.6g; Cholesterol: 12mg; Sodium: 67mg

11.Steamed French and Broad Beans

Yield: 6 Servings, Prep Time: 5 Minutes, Cook Time: 18 Minutes

Ingredients

- 1 cup French beans, washed
- 1 cup broad beans, washed
- 1 teaspoon ginger powder
- 3 cups water
- 3 tablespoons olive oil
- Salt and black pepper, to taste

Directions:

1. Season the French beans and broad beans with ginger powder, salt and black pepper
2. Place the steamer trivet in the bottom of Instant Pot and add water.
3. Put the seasoned beans on the trivet.
4. Set the Instant Pot to "Manual" at high pressure for 12 minutes.
5. Release the pressure naturally and remove the trivet.
6. Put the olive oil and beans and select "Sauté".
7. Sauté for 5 minutes and stir in the lemon juice.

Nutritional Information per Serving:

Calories: 260; Total Fat: 8g; Carbs: 37.2g; Sugars: 0.7g; Protein: 11.1g; Cholesterol: 0mg; Sodium: 13mg

12.Delicious Succotash

Yield: 6 Servings, Prep Time: 7 Minutes, Cook Time: 13 Minutes

Ingredients

- 1 cup bell peppers
- 2 cups complete corn kernels
- 2 cups water
- 3 tablespoons butter
- 2 cups lima beans
- 2 cups tomatoes
- 2 teaspoons salt

Directions:

1. Put the butter and bell peppers in the Instant Pot and select "Sauté".
2. Sauté for 3 minutes and add rest of the ingredients.
3. Set the Instant Pot to "Manual" at high pressure for 10 minutes.
4. Release the pressure naturally and serve hot.

Nutritional Information per Serving:

Calories: 153; Total Fat: 6.7g; Carbs: 19.7g; Sugars: 5.4g; Protein: 5g; Cholesterol: 15mg; Sodium: 929mg

13. Vegetable Medley

Yield: 3 Servings, Prep Time: 5 Minutes, Cook Time: 9 Minutes

Ingredients

- 1 small sweet potato, peeled and diced
- 2 carrots, peeled and diced
- 3 pink potatoes, quartered
- 1½ cups butternut squash
- 1 tablespoon olive oil
- 1 sprig rosemary
- ½ cup water
- Salt and pepper, to taste

Directions:

1. Put the olive oil and rosemary sprig in the Instant Pot and select "Sauté".
2. Sauté for 2 minutes and add rest of the ingredients.
3. Set the Instant Pot to "Manual" at high pressure for 7 minutes.
4. Release the pressure naturally and serve hot.

Nutritional Information per Serving:

Calories: 202; Total Fat: 5.2g; Carbs: 40.6g; Sugars: 9g; Protein: 3.6g; Cholesterol: 0mg; Sodium: 48mg

14.Spicy Cauliflower

Yield: 3 Servings, Prep Time: 10 Minutes, Cook Time: 5 Minutes

Ingredients

- 1 pound cauliflower
- ½ cup vegetable broth
- 1 tablespoon fresh lemon juice
- 1 tablespoon olive oil
- 1 teaspoon red pepper flakes, crushed
- Salt, to taste

Directions:

1. Season the cauliflower with salt and red pepper flakes.
2. Put the olive oil and cauliflowers in the Instant Pot and select "Sauté".
3. Sauté for 4 minutes and add vegetable broth.
4. Set the Instant Pot to "Manual" at high pressure for 6 minutes.
5. Release the pressure naturally and stir in the lemon juice.

Nutritional Information per Serving:

Calories: 87; Total Fat: 5.2g; Carbs: 8.6g; Sugars: 3.9g; Protein: 3.9g; Cholesterol: 0mg; Sodium: 174mg

15.Nutty Brussels Sprouts

Yield: 3 Servings, Prep Time: 5 Minutes, Cook Time: 4 Minutes

Ingredients

- 1 pound brussels sprouts, trimmed and halved
- ½ tablespoon butter, melted
- ½ cup almonds, chopped
- 1 teaspoon salt

Directions:

1. Place the steamer trivet in the bottom of Instant Pot and add water.
2. Put the brussels sprouts on the trivet.
3. Set the Instant Pot to "Manual" at high pressure for 4 minutes.
4. Release the pressure quickly and remove the trivet.
5. Drizzle with butter and top with almonds.

Nutritional Information per Serving:

Calories: 174; Total Fat: 10.4g; Carbs: 17.1g; Sugars: 3.9g; Protein: 8.5g; Cholesterol: 5mg; Sodium: 52mg

16.Simple Broccoli

Yield: 3 Servings, Prep Time: 5 Minutes, Cook Time: 5 Minutes

Ingredients

- 1 pound broccoli florets
- 1 cup water
- 2 tablespoons butter, melted
- Salt and freshly ground black pepper, to taste

Directions:

1. Place the steamer trivet in the bottom of Instant Pot and add water.
2. Put the broccoli florets on the trivet.
3. Set the Instant Pot to "Manual" at high pressure for 5 minutes.
4. Release the pressure quickly and remove the trivet.
5. Drizzle with butter and season with salt and black pepper.

Nutritional Information per Serving:

Calories: 119; Total Fat: 8.2g; Carbs: 10.1g; Sugars: 2.6g; Protein: 4.3g; Cholesterol: 20mg; Sodium: 104mg

17.Refreshing Green Beans

Yield: 6 Servings, Prep Time: 5 Minutes, Cook Time: 6 Minutes

Ingredients

- 2 pounds fresh green beans
- 2 garlic cloves, minced
- 4 tablespoons butter
- 3 cups water
- Salt and freshly ground black pepper, to taste

Directions:

1. Put the fresh green beans and all other ingredients in the Instant Pot.
2. Set the Instant Pot to "Manual" at high pressure for 6 minutes.
3. Release the pressure quickly and serve hot.

Nutritional Information per Serving:

Calories: 116; Total Fat: 7.9g; Carbs: 11.1g; Sugars: 2.1g; Protein: 2.9g; Cholesterol: 20mg; Sodium: 64mg

18.Kale and Carrots Platter

Yield: 4 Servings, Prep Time: 5 Minutes, Cook Time: 17 Minutes

Ingredients

- 1 cup fresh kale, trimmed and chopped
- 3 medium carrots, peeled and cut into ½-inch slices
- 5 garlic cloves, minced
- 2tablespoons olive oil
- 1 small onion, chopped
- ½ cup vegetable broth
- 1 tablespoon fresh lemon juice
- ¼ teaspoon red pepper flakes, crushed
- Salt and black pepper, to taste

Directions:

1. Put the olive oil, garlic and onions in the Instant Pot and select "Sauté".
2. Sauté for 4 minutes and add carrots.
3. Sauté for 3 minutes and add broth, kale, red pepper flakes, salt and black pepper.
4. Set the Instant Pot to "Manual" at high pressure for 9 minutes.
5. Release the pressure naturally and stir in the lemon juice.

Nutritional Information per Serving:

Calories: 103; Total Fat: 7.1g; Carbs: 9.7g; Sugars: 3.4g; Protein: 1.4g; Cholesterol: 0mg; Sodium: 107mg

19.Healthy Spinach Plate

Yield: 3 Servings, Prep Time: 5 Minutes, Cook Time: 14 Minutes

Ingredients

- 5 cups fresh spinach, chopped
- 1 small onion, chopped
- 1 cup vegetable broth
- 1 tablespoon garlic, minced
- 1tablespoon olive oil
- 1 tablespoon fresh lemon juice
- ½ cup tomatoes, chopped
- ½ cup tomato puree
- ½ teaspoon red pepper flakes, crushed
- Salt and freshly ground black pepper, to taste

Directions:

1. Put the olive oil, garlic and onions in the Instant Pot and select "Sauté".
2. Sauté for 4 minutes and add spinach, red pepper flakes, salt and black pepper.
3. Sauté for 3 minutes and add in the remaining ingredients.
4. Set the Instant Pot to "Manual" at high pressure for 7 minutes.
5. Release the pressure quickly and serve hot.

Nutritional Information per Serving:

Calories: 101 ; Total Fat: 5.6g; Carbs: 10.4g; Sugars: 4.4g; Protein: 4.5g; Cholesterol: 0mg; Sodium: 310mg

20.Colorful Veggies

Yield: 8 Servings, Prep Time: 5 Minutes, Cook Time: 13 Minutes

Ingredients

- 2 tablespoons olive oil
- 3 garlic cloves, minced
- 3 small yellow onions, chopped roughly
- 1½ pounds cherry tomatoes
- 8 medium zucchinis, chopped roughly
- 1½ cups water
- 3 tablespoons fresh basil, chopped
- Salt and black pepper, to taste

Directions:

1. Put the olive oil, garlic and onions in the Instant Pot and select "Sauté". Sauté for 4 minutes.
2. Add zucchinis and tomatoes. Sauté for 3 minutes, then add water. Set the Instant Pot to "Manual" at high pressure for 6 minutes.
3. Release the pressure naturally and add salt, black pepper.
4. Garnish with basil, serve and enjoy.

Nutritional Information per Serving:

Calories: 130; Total Fat: 4.5g; Carbs: 21.6g; Sugars: 12.7g; Protein: 5.5g; Cholesterol: 0mg; Sodium: 41mg

DELICIOUS VEGETARIAN SOUP RECIPES

21.Basil Tomato Soup

Yield: 4 Servings , Prep Time: 10 Minutes, Cook Time: 20 Minutes

Ingredients

- 1 garlic clove, minced
- 1 tablespoon olive oil
- 1 medium onion, chopped
- 3 pounds fresh tomatoes, chopped
- 2 teaspoons dried parsley, crushed
- 2 tablespoons homemade tomato sauce

- 4 cups low-sodium vegetable broth
- Freshly ground black pepper, to taste
- 2 tablespoons sugar
- 1 tablespoon balsamic vinegar
- ¼ cup fresh basil, chopped

Directions

1. Put the oil, garlic and onion in the Instant Pot and select "Sauté", sauté for 4 minutes.
2. Add the parsley, tomatoes, tomato sauce, broth and black pepper, cook for about 3 minutes and lock the lid.
3. Set the Instant Pot to "Soup" and cook for 10 minutes at high pressure.
4. Release the pressure quickly and stir in the vinegar and sugar.
5. Put the mixture in the immersion blender and puree the soup.
6. Garnish with basil and serve.

Nutritional Information per Serving:

Calories: 146; Total Fat: 4.5 g; Carbs: 23.5 g; Sugars: 16.4 g; Protein: 5.4 g; Cholesterol: 0 mg; Sodium: 110mg

22.Tarragon Corn Soup

Yield: 4 Servings, Prep Time: 10 Minutes, Cook Time: 5 Minutes

Ingredients

- 2 tablespoons butter
- 2 medium garlic cloves, thinly sliced
- 2 bay leaves
- 6 corn with cobs, cut in halves
- 4 sprigs Tarragon
- 1 tablespoon chives, minced
- Salt and black pepper, to taste

Directions:

1. Put the butter, garlic in the Instant Pot and select "Sauté". Sauté for 4 minutes.
2. Add the bay leaves, corn with cobs, and tarragon sprigs, then add water to cover food up 1/2 inch.
3. Set the Instant Pot to "Soup" and cook for 10 minutes at high pressure.
4. Release the pressure quickly and discard bay leaf and tarragon sprigs.
5. Season the corn soup with salt and black pepper and simmer for 3 minutes.
6. Add the chives and sever.

Nutritional Information per Serving:

Calories: 323; Total Fat: 11.5g; Carbs: 55.8g; Sugars: 2.38g; Protein: 8.3g; Cholesterol: 24mg; Sodium: 667mg

23.Corn and Potato Soup

Yield: 4 Servings, Prep Time: 10 Minutes, Cook Time: 17 Minutes

Ingredients

- 2 cups fresh corn kernels
- 2 large russet potatoes, peeled and chopped
- 2 tablespoons butter
- 2 celery stalks, chopped
- 2 garlic cloves, chopped finely
- 1 teaspoon black pepper, freshly ground
- 6 cups low-sodium vegetable broth
- 3 tablespoons corn-starch
- ¼ cup half-and-half
- 3 carrots, peeled and chopped
- 1 medium onion, chopped
- 2 tablespoons dried parsley, crushed

Directions:

1. Put the butter, carrot, celery, garlic and onions in the Instant Pot and select "Sauté".
2. Sauté for 4 minutes and add corn kernels, potatoes, broth, parsley and black pepper.
3. Set the Instant Pot to "Soup" and cook for 10 minutes at high pressure.
4. Release the pressure quickly and open the lid.
5. Dissolve the corn starch in half-and-half and add to the Instant Pot.
6. Select "Sauté" and cook for about 3 minutes.

Nutritional Information per Serving:

Calories: 343; Total Fat: 8.7g; Carbs: 59.1g; Sugars: 8.2g; Protein: 10g; Cholesterol: 21mg; Sodium: 216mg

24.Creamy Broccoli Soup

Yield: 3 Servings, Prep Time: 5 Minutes, Cook Time: 17 Minutes

Ingredients

- 1 cup broccoli florets, washed and blanched
- 2 garlic cloves, minced
- 2tablespoons butter
- 1 teaspoon black pepper, freshly ground
- ½ cup full fat milk
- 1 small onion, chopped
- 1 tablespoon celery leaves, chopped
- 1 teaspoon salt
- ½ cup cream
- 1 cup vegetable stock

Directions:

1. Put the butter, celery, garlic and onions in the Instant Pot and select "Sauté".
2. Sauté for 4 minutes and add broccoli florets, vegetable stock, salt and black pepper.
3. Set the Instant Pot to "Soup" and cook for 10 minutes at high pressure.
4. Release the pressure quickly and open the lid.
5. Put the mixture in the blender and add milk and cream.
6. Put back in the Instant Pot and let it simmer for 3 minutes.

Nutritional Information per Serving:

Calories: 134; Total Fat: 10.1g; Carbs: 8.9g; Sugars: 4.6g; Protein: 3.4g; Cholesterol: 29mg; Sodium: 894mg

25. Creamy Mushroom Soup

Yield: 4 Servings, Prep Time: 10 Minutes, Cook Time: 15 Minutes

Ingredients

- 10 oz. cremini mushrooms, thinly sliced
- 1 tablespoon olive oil
- 3 garlic cloves, minced
- 2 carrots, peeled and diced
- ½ teaspoon dried thyme
- ½ cup half-and-half
- 2 tablespoons fresh parsley leaves, chopped
- 2 tablespoons butter
- 1 onion, diced
- 2 stalks celery, diced
- ¼ cup all-purpose flour
- 1 bay leaf
- 1 sprig rosemary

Directions:

1. Put the olive oil, mushrooms, carrot, butter, celery, garlic, thyme and onions in the Instant Pot and select "Sauté".

2. Sauté for 4 minutes and add in the flour until light brown.

3. Add bay leaf and close the lid.

4. Set the Instant Pot to "Soup" and cook for 10 minutes at high pressure.

5. Release the pressure quickly and add half and half.

6. Season with salt and black pepper and garnish with rosemary and parsley.

Nutritional Information per Serving:

Calories: 208; Total Fat: 13.6g; Carbs: 18g; Sugars: 4.8g; Protein: 5.1g; Cholesterol: 26mg; Sodium: 852mg

26.Pumpkin and Tomato Soup

Yield: 4 Servings, Prep Time: 10 Minutes, Cook Time: 5 Minutes

Ingredients

- 4 tablespoons pumpkin puree
- 1 cup tomatoes, chopped
- 4 tablespoons butter
- 1 carrot, roughly chopped
- 1 potato, roughly diced
- 3 tablespoons sun dried tomatoes
- 4 cups water
- 1 onion, roughly sliced
- 3 tablespoons tomato paste
- 1 teaspoon pumpkin spice powder
- 2 teaspoons salt
- 2 pinches black pepper

Directions:

1. Put the butter, carrots and onions in the Instant Pot and select "Sauté".
2. Sauté for 4 minutes and add potatoes, tomatoes, tomato paste, sun dried tomatoes, pumpkin puree, water, salt and black pepper.
3. Set the Instant Pot to "Soup" and cook for 15 minutes at high pressure.
4. Release the pressure naturally and add blend the mixture to a smooth consistency.
5. Sprinkle pumpkin spice powder and serve.

Nutritional Information per Serving:

Calories: 190; Total Fat: 12.7g; Carbs: 18.5g; Sugars: 5.9g; Protein: 2.8g; Cholesterol: 31mg; Sodium: 1296mg

27.Spinach Cream Soup

Yield: 3 Servings, Prep Time: 5 Minutes, Cook Time: 15 Minutes

Ingredients

- 1 cup spinach puree
- ½ cup fresh cream
- 3tablespoons butter
- 1 cup white sauce
- 3 garlic cloves, minced
- 1 medium onion, roughly sliced
- 1 tablespoon tomato paste
- 1 tablespoon sun dried tomatoes
- 4 cups water
- 2 teaspoons salt
- 2 pinches black pepper

Directions:

1. Put the butter, garlic, salt, black pepper and onions in the Instant Pot and select "Sauté".
2. Sauté for 4 minutes and add water, spinach puree and tomato paste.
3. Set the Instant Pot to "Soup" and cook for 10 minutes at high pressure.
4. Release the pressure naturally and add fresh cream and white sauce.
5. Blend the contents of the Instant Pot to a smooth consistency and garnish with sun dried tomatoes.

Nutritional Information per Serving:

Calories: 305; Total Fat: 23.7g; Carbs: 17.6g; Sugars: 6.7g; Protein: 5.9g; Cholesterol: 44mg; Sodium: 2103mg

28. Sour Cream Black Beans Soup

Yield: 3 Servings, Prep Time: 7 Minutes, Cook Time: 13 Minutes

Ingredients

- 1 cup black beans
- 5 garlic cloves, minced
- 3 tablespoons tomato paste
- ¼ cup sour cream
- 4 cups water
- 3 tablespoons butter
- 1 onion, roughly sliced
- 1 potato, roughly diced
- 1 tablespoon sun dried tomatoes
- 2 tablespoons fresh cream
- 2 teaspoons salt
- 2 pinches black pepper
- Crunchy nachos chips, for garnish

Directions:

1. Put the butter, garlic and onions in the Instant Pot and select "Sauté".
2. Sauté for 3 minutes and add black beans, tomato paste, water, sun dried tomatoes, salt and black pepper.
3. Set the Instant Pot to "Soup" and cook for 10 minutes at high pressure.
4. Release the pressure naturally and add sour cream.
5. Blend the contents of the Instant Pot to a smooth consistency and serve with fresh cream and broken nachos chips.

Nutritional Information per Serving:

Calories: 339; Total Fat: 13.1g; Carbs: 45g; Sugars: 4.2g; Protein: 13.1g; Cholesterol: 30mg; Sodium: 1264mg

29.Basil Tomato Soup

Yield: 2 Servings, Prep Time: 5 Minutes, Cook Time: 12 Minutes

Ingredients

- ½ cup tomatoes
- 2 tablespoons tomato paste
- 2 tablespoons sun dried tomatoes
- 2tablespoons butter
- 1tablespoon basil leaves, freshly chopped
- 1 carrot, roughly chopped
- 1 onion, roughly sliced
- 1 potato, roughly diced
- 4 cups water
- 2 teaspoons salt
- ¼ teaspoon black pepper

Directions:

1. Put the butter, onions, carrots, basil leaves, salt and black pepper in the Instant Pot and select "Sauté".
2. Sauté for 4 minutes and add potatoes, tomatoes, sun dried tomatoes, tomato paste and water.
3. Set the Instant Pot to "Soup" and cook for 8 minutes at high pressure.
4. Release the pressure naturally and blend the contents of the Instant Pot to a smooth consistency.

Nutritional Information per Serving:

Calories: 239; Total Fat: 12.8g; Carbs: 29.6g; Sugars: 7.6g; Protein: 4.2g; Cholesterol: 31mg; Sodium: 2486mg

30.Chestnut Soup

Yield: 4 Servings, Prep Time: 10 Minutes, Cook Time: 15 Minutes

Ingredients

- ½ pound fresh chestnuts
- 4 tablespoons butter
- 1 sprig sage
- ¼ teaspoon white pepper
- ¼ teaspoon nutmeg
- 1 onion, chopped
- 1 stalk celery, chopped
- 1 potato, chopped
- 2 tablespoons rum
- 2 tablespoons fresh cream

Directions:

1. Puree the fresh chestnuts in a blender.
2. Put the butter, onions, sage, celery and white pepper in the Instant Pot and select "Sauté".
3. Sauté for 4 minutes and add potato, stock and chestnuts.
4. Set the Instant Pot to "Soup" and cook for 15 minutes at high pressure.
5. Release the pressure naturally and add rum, nutmeg and fresh cream.
6. Blend the contents of the Instant Pot to a smooth consistency.

Nutritional Information per Serving:

Calories: 290; Total Fat: 13.3g; Carbs: 36.5g; Sugars: 2.5g; Protein: 3g; Cholesterol: 32mg; Sodium: 856mg

31.Tortilla and White Beans Soup

Yield: 4 Servings, Prep Time: 10 Minutes, Cook Time: 17 Minutes

Ingredients

- 1 cup white beans
- 4 tablespoons butter
- ¼ teaspoon white pepper
- 1 onion, roughly sliced
- 1 tablespoon sun dried tomatoes
- ¼ cup fresh cream
- 4 cups water
- 2 teaspoons salt
- 1 carrot, roughly chopped
- 4 garlic cloves, minced
- 4 tablespoons tomato paste
- Crunchy tortilla chips, for garnish

Directions:

1. Put the butter, garlic, carrots, onions and white pepper in the Instant Pot and select "Sauté".
2. Sauté for 5 minutes and add white beans, potatoes, sun dried tomatoes, tomato paste, salt and water.
3. Set the Instant Pot to "Soup" and cook for 12 minutes at high pressure.
4. Release the pressure naturally and add sour cream.
5. Blend the contents of the Instant Pot to a smooth consistency and top with crunchy tortilla chips.

Nutritional Information per Serving:

Calories: 353; Total Fat: 14.7g; Carbs: 44.2g; Sugars: 5.3g; Protein: 14g; Cholesterol: 33mg; Sodium: 1337mg

32.Vegetable Noodle Soup

Yield: 5 Servings, Prep Time: 8 Minutes, Cook Time: 12 Minutes

Ingredients

- ½ cup potatoes, diced
- ½ cup peas
- ½ cup carrots
- ½ cup cauliflower
- 6 oz. noodles, cooked and drained
- ½ cup onions
- 3 garlic cloves, minced
- ½ inch ginger, minced

- 1 cup tomatoes, diced
- 10 oz. baby carrots
- 2 teaspoons Worcestershire sauce
- 32 oz. vegetable stock
- 1 tablespoon olive oil
- 1 teaspoon salt
- 1 teaspoon black pepper

Directions:

1. Put the oil, ginger, garlic, carrots, onions and cauliflowers in the Instant Pot and select "Sauté".
2. Sauté for 5 minutes and add potatoes, tomatoes, peas, vegetable stock and Worcestershire sauce.
3. Set the Instant Pot to "Soup" and cook for 12 minutes at high pressure.
4. Release the pressure naturally and add cooked noodles.
5. Season with salt and black pepper and serve immediately.

Nutritional Information per Serving:

Calories: 148; Total Fat: 4g; Carbs: 24.8g; Sugars: 7.8g; Protein: 4.6g; Cholesterol: 10mg; Sodium: 174mg

33.Manchow Soup

Yield: 4 Servings, Prep Time: 10 Minutes, Cook Time: 15 Minutes

Ingredients

- 3 oz. fried noodles, for garnish
- ½ cup green bell peppers
- ½ cup bean sprouts
- ½ cup mushrooms
- ½ cup broccoli
- ½ cup baby carrots
- 2 green onions, chopped
- 4 garlic cloves, minced

- ½ inch ginger, minced
- 1 teaspoon soy sauce
- 1 teaspoon vinegar
- 2 teaspoons chilli sauce
- 3 cups vegetable stock
- 1 tablespoon oil
- Salt and pepper, to taste
- Roasted crushed peanuts, for garnish

Directions:

1. Put the oil, ginger, garlic, carrots, onions and carrots in the Instant Pot and select "Sauté".
2. Sauté for 4 minutes and add soy sauce, chilli sauce, vinegar and vegetable stock.
3. Set the Instant Pot to "Soup" and cook for 10 minutes at high pressure.
4. Release the pressure naturally and add cooked noodles.
5. Season with salt and black pepper and garnish with fried noodles and crushed roasted peanuts.

Nutritional Information per Serving:

Calories: 379; Total Fat: 20.8g; Carbs: 43.6g; Sugars: 2.4g; Protein: 8.7g; Cholesterol: 0mg; Sodium: 425mg

34.Chinese Noodle Soup

Yield: 8 Servings, Prep Time: 10 Minutes, Cook Time: 20 Minutes

Ingredients

- 12 oz. noodles, cooked and drained
- 1 cup red bell peppers
- 1 cup mushrooms
- 1 cup broccoli
- 1 cup bokchoy
- 4 green onion whites
- 8 garlic cloves, minced
- 1 inch ginger, minced
- 2 teaspoons soy sauce
- 1 teaspoon white chilli vinegar
- 20 oz. baby carrots
- 2 teaspoons chilli sauce
- 8 cups vegetable stock
- 2 tablespoons oil
- Salt and pepper, to taste
- Onion greens, for garnish

Directions:

1. Put the oil, ginger, garlic, baby carrots and onions in the Instant Pot and select "Sauté".
2. Sauté for 4 minutes and add broccoli, bokchoy, red bell peppers, mushrooms, soy sauce, chilli vinegar, chilli sauce and vegetable stock.
3. Set the Instant Pot to "Soup" and cook for 15 minutes at high pressure.
4. Release the pressure naturally and add cooked noodles.
5. Season with salt and black pepper and garnish with onion greens.

Nutritional Information per Serving:

Calories: 145; Total Fat: 4.7g; Carbs: 22.6g; Sugars: 6.1g; Protein: 4g; Cholesterol: 12mg; Sodium: 207mg

35.Japanese Udon Noodle Soup

Yield: 2 Servings, Prep Time: 10 Minutes, Cook Time: 17 Minutes

Ingredients

- 3 oz. Japanese udon noodles, cooked and drained
- ½ cup green bell peppers
- ½ cup celery
- ½ cup mushrooms
- ½ cup bamboo shoots
- 2 garlic cloves, minced
- ½ green chilli, finely chopped
- ½ cup baby carrots
- 1 teaspoon rice vinegar soy sauce
- ½ inch ginger, minced
- 1 green onion white
- 1 teaspoon rice wine vinegar
- 1 teaspoon red chilli sauce
- 1 tablespoon sesame oil
- Bean sprouts and green onions, for garnish
- Salt and pepper, to taste

Directions:

1. Put the oil, ginger, garlic, baby carrots and onions in the Instant Pot and select "Sauté".
2. Sauté for 4 minutes and add bamboo shoots, celery, green bell peppers, mushrooms, soy sauce, rice wine vinegar, chilli sauce.
3. Set the Instant Pot to "Soup" and cook for 13 minutes at high pressure.
4. Release the pressure naturally and add cooked udon noodles.
5. Season with salt and black pepper and garnish with onion greens and bean sprouts.

Nutritional Information per Serving:

Calories: 179; Total Fat: 3.9g; Carbs: 30g; Sugars: 2.7g; Protein: 3.6g; Cholesterol: 0mg; Sodium: 473mg

36.Pearl Barley Soup

Yield: 6 Servings, Prep Time: 8 Minutes, Cook Time: 18 Minutes

Ingredients

- 1 cup all-purpose flour
- 2 onions, chopped
- 2 celery stalks, chopped
- 2 carrots, chopped
- 4 tablespoons olive oil
- 2 cups mushroom, sliced
- 28 oz. vegetable stock
- ¾ cup pearl barley
- 2 teaspoons dried oregano
- 1 cup purple wine
- Salt and pepper, to taste

Directions:

1. Put the oil, garlic and onions in the Instant Pot and select "Sauté".
2. Sauté for 3 minutes and add rest of the ingredients.
3. Set the Instant Pot to "Soup" and cook for 15 minutes at high pressure.
4. Release the pressure naturally and serve hot.

Nutritional Information per Serving:

Calories: 310; Total Fat: 10.1g; Carbs: 43.8g; Sugars: 4.2g; Protein: 6.6g; Cholesterol: 0mg; Sodium: 92mg

37.Lemon Rice Soup

Yield: 6 Servings, Prep Time: 10 Minutes, Cook Time: 16 Minutes

Ingredients

- ¾ cup lengthy grain rice
- 1 cup onions, sliced
- 1 cup carrots, chopped
- 6 cups vegetable broth
- Salt and pepper, to taste
- ¾ cup lemon juice, freshly squeezed
- 3 teaspoons minced garlic
- 1 cup celery, chopped
- 2 tablespoons olive oil
- 2 tablespoons all-purpose flour

Directions:

1. Put the oil, garlic, celery and onions in the Instant Pot and select "Sauté".
2. Sauté for 4 minutes and add rest of the ingredients except all-purpose flour and lemon juice.
3. Set the Instant Pot to "Soup" and cook for 12 minutes at high pressure.
4. Release the pressure naturally and add the whisked lemon juice+ all-purpose flour mixture.
5. Let it simmer till the soup becomes thick and season with salt and pepper.

Nutritional Information per Serving:

Calories: 225; Total Fat: 12g; Carbs: 25.5g; Sugars: 4.9g; Protein: 5.1g; Cholesterol: 2mg; Sodium: 1032mg

38.Basil Coriander Lemon Soup

Yield: 3 Servings, Prep Time: 10 Minutes, Cook Time: 17 Minutes

Ingredients

- ½ cup onions, sliced
- ½ cup carrots, chopped
- 16 oz. can vegetable broth
- 1/3 cup fresh coriander, chopped
- ¼ cup lemon juice, freshly squeezed
- 2 teaspoons garlic, minced
- ½ cup celery, chopped
- 2 tablespoons olive oil
- 1/3 cup fresh basil leaves, chopped
- Salt and pepper, to taste
- 2 tablespoons all-purpose flour

Directions:

1. Put the oil, garlic, celery and onions in the Instant Pot and select "Sauté".
2. Sauté for 4 minutes and add rest of the ingredients except all-purpose flour and lemon juice.
3. Set the Instant Pot to "Soup" and cook for 13 minutes at high pressure.
4. Release the pressure naturally and add the whisked lemon juice and all-purpose flour mixture.
5. Let it simmer till the soup becomes thick and season with salt and pepper.

Nutritional Information per Serving:

Calories: 135; Total Fat: 9.6g; Carbs: 11.2g; Sugars: 3.7g; Protein: 1.4g; Cholesterol: 0mg; Sodium: 366mg

39.Beetroot Soup

Yield: 4 Servings, Prep Time: 10 Minutes, Cook Time: 20 Minutes

Ingredients

- 2 pounds beetroot, peeled and diced
- 3 teaspoons garlic, minced
- ½ cup onions, sliced
- ½ cup celery, chopped
- ½ cup carrots, chopped
- 3 tablespoons olive oil
- 4 cups vegetable broth
- 3 tablespoons fresh coriander, chopped
- Salt and pepper, to taste
- 3 tablespoons fresh cream

Directions:

1. Put the oil, garlic, celery and onions in the Instant Pot and select "Sauté".
2. Sauté for 4 minutes and add rest of the ingredients except fresh cream.
3. Set the Instant Pot to "Soup" and cook for 16 minutes at high pressure.
4. Release the pressure naturally and add the fresh cream.
5. Season with salt and pepper and garnish with coriander leaves.

Nutritional Information per Serving:

Calories: 251; Total Fat: 12.8g; Carbs: 27.6g; Sugars: 20.4g; Protein: 9.2g;
Cholesterol: 2mg; Sodium: 962mg

40.Lentil and Smoked Paprika Soup

Yield: 10 Servings, Prep Time: 10 Minutes, Cook Time: 11 Minutes

Ingredients

- 2 cups red lentils, rinsed
- 2cups green lentils, rinse
- 1½ pounds potatoes
- 1½ bunches rainbow chard
- 2 onions, chopped finely
- 4 teaspoons cumin
- 2teaspoons salt
- 2 celery stalks
- 6 garlic cloves, minced
- 3 teaspoons smoked paprika
- 4 carrots, sliced
- 10 cups water
- Salt and pepper, to taste

Directions:

1. Put the oil, garlic, celery and onions in the Instant Pot and select "Sauté".
2. Sauté for 4 minutes and add rest of the ingredients except lentils.
3. Set the Instant Pot to "Soup" and cook for 7 minutes at high pressure.
4. Release the pressure naturally and add season with salt and pepper.

Nutritional Information per Serving:

Calories: 209; Total Fat: 0.8g; Carbs: 39.6g; Sugars: 3.9g; Protein: 11.9g; Cholesterol: 0mg; Sodium: 501mg

FLAVORFUL RICE, BEANS AND LENTILS RECIPES

41.Kidney Beans with Veggies

Yield: 4 Servings, Prep Time: 10 Minutes, Cook Time: 45 Minutes

Ingredients

- 1 cup kidney beans, soaked overnight
- 1 medium carrot, chopped
- 1 cup tomatoes, chopped
- 3 tablespoons fresh basil
- 1 teaspoon thyme
- 1teaspoon red pepper flakes
- 1 small onion, sliced
- 3 garlic cloves, minced
- 1 tablespoon olive oil
- 1 teaspoon oregano
- Salt and black pepper, to taste

Directions:

1. Put the olive oil, garlic and onions in the Instant Pot and select "Sauté".
2. Sauté for 4 minutes and add red pepper flakes, oregano, fresh basil, thyme, salt and black pepper.
3. Sauté for 1 minute and add tomatoes, carrots, water and kidney beans.
4. Set the Instant Pot to "Manual" at high pressure for 40 minutes.
5. Release the pressure quickly and dish out.

Nutritional Information per Serving:

Calories: 213; Total Fat: 4.3g; Carbs: 34.5g; Sugars: 3.7g; Protein: 11.4g; Cholesterol: 0mg; Sodium: 20mg

42.Parsley in Chickpeas

Yield: 3 Servings, Prep Time: 10 Minutes, Cook Time: 25 Minutes

Ingredients

- ½ cup chickpeas, soaked overnight
- 4 cups water
- 1 small onion, sliced
- 2 garlic cloves, minced
- 2 tablespoons olive oil
- ¼ cup parsley, chopped
- ¼ cup dill leaves, chopped
- 2 tablespoons fresh lemon juice
- 1 teaspoon salt

Directions:

1. Put water and chickpeas in the Instant Pot.
2. Set the Instant Pot to "Manual" at high pressure for 25 minutes.
3. Release the pressure naturally and put the mixture in a blender.
4. Add rest of the ingredients and blend thoroughly.

Nutritional Information per Serving:

Calories: 228; Total Fat: 11.7g; Carbs: 25.8g; Sugars: 4.8g; Protein: 7.9g; Cholesterol: 0mg; Sodium: 32mg

43.Kidney Beans Curry

Yield: 3 Servings, Prep Time: 10 Minutes, Cook Time: 25 Minutes

Ingredients

- 1 cup dried red kidney beans, soaked for overnight and drained
- ¼ cup split chickpeas, soaked for overnight and drained
- 4 cups water
- 3 tablespoons olive oil
- 3 teaspoons garlic, minced
- 1 large tomato, chopped finely
- 2 medium onions, chopped
- 3 teaspoons fresh ginger, minced
- 1½ teaspoons ground coriander
- 1½ teaspoons ground turmeric
- 1½ teaspoons ground cumin
- 2 teaspoons red chilli powder
- ¼ teaspoon salt
- 4 tablespoons fresh cilantro, chopped

Directions:

1. Put the olive oil, garlic, ginger and onions in the Instant Pot and select "Sauté".
2. Sauté for 4 minutes and add ground coriander, ground turmeric, ground cumin, red chilli powder and salt.
3. Sauté for 4 minutes and add water, tomatoes, beans and split chickpeas
4. Set the Instant Pot to "Manual" at high pressure for 20 minutes.
5. Release the pressure naturally and garnish with fresh cilantro.

Nutritional Information per Serving:

Calories: 427; Total Fat: 17.5g; Carbs: 64.4g; Sugars: 8.2g; Protein: 20g; Cholesterol: 0mg; Sodium: 247mg

44.Chickpeas Curry

Yield: 6 Servings, Prep Time: 10 Minutes, Cook Time: 25 Minutes

Ingredients

- 2 cups dried chickpeas, soaked overnight
- 4 medium tomatoes, chopped finely
- 2 tablespoons olive oil
- 2 onions, chopped
- 4 cups water
- 2 tablespoons fresh ginger, minced
- 2 tablespoons garlic, minced
- 2 teaspoons curry powder
- 2 teaspoons ground cumin
- 1 teaspoon ground coriander
- ½ teaspoon salt
- ½ teaspoon black pepper, to taste
- ½ cup fresh parsley, chopped

Directions:

1. Put the oil and onions in the Instant Pot and select "Sauté".
2. Sauté for 3 minutes and add garlic, ginger, curry powder, ground cumin, ground coriander, salt and black pepper.
3. Sauté for 2 minutes and add tomatoes, chickpeas and water.
4. Set the Instant Pot to "Manual" at high pressure for 20 minutes.
5. Release the pressure naturally and garnish with parsley.

Nutritional Information per Serving:

Calories: 330; Total Fat: 9.3g; Carbs: 50.4g; Sugars: 11g; Protein: 14.7g; Cholesterol: 0mg; Sodium: 226mg

45.Quinoa Pilaf

Yield: 8 Servings, Prep Time: 5 Minutes, Cook Time: 3 Minutes

Ingredients

- 3 cups quinoa, rinsed and drained
- 2 tablespoons butter
- 1 cup onions, chopped
- 1 cup almonds, sliced
- ½ cup dried cherries
- ½ cup water
- 2 celery stalks, chopped finely

Directions

1. Put the butter, celery, garlic and onions in the Instant Pot and select "Sauté".
2. Sauté for 4 minutes and add rest of the ingredients except almonds.
3. Set the Instant Pot to "Manual" at high pressure for 2 minutes.
4. Release the pressure quickly and stir in the almonds.

Nutritional Information per Serving:

Calories: 388; Total Fat: 13.1g; Carbs: 55.6g; Sugars: 1.3g; Protein: 13.1g; Cholesterol: 8mg; Sodium: 226mg

46.Green Gram Lentil Curry

Yield: 4 Servings, Prep Time: 5 Minutes, Cook Time: 20 Minutes

Ingredients

- 1½cups green gram lentils whole, rinsed
- 1tablespoon garlic, minced
- 1½ tablespoons lemon juice
- 1½ tablespoons ginger, minced
- 4 cups water
- 1½ teaspoons salt
- 1½ teaspoons cumin seeds
- 3 medium tomatoes, chopped
- 1½tablespoons oil
- 2 medium onions, diced
- Cilantro, to garnish

Directions:

1. Put the oil, cumin seeds, garlic and onions in the Instant Pot and select "Sauté".
2. Sauté for 4 minutes and add tomato, lentils, water and spices.
3. Set the instant pot to "Manual" and cook for 15 minutes at high pressure.
4. Release the pressure naturally and add lime juice and cilantro.

Nutritional Information per Serving:

Calories: 354; Total Fat: 6.5g; Carbs: 54.8g; Sugars: 6.5g; Protein: 20.6g; Cholesterol: 0mg; Sodium: 896mg

47.Chickpea, White Bean and Tomato Stew

Yield: 4 Servings, Prep Time: 10 Minutes, Cook Time: 30 Minutes

Ingredients

- 1 cup dried white beans, soaked overnight
- 1 cup dried chickpeas, soaked overnight
- ¼ cup dried red lentils
- 1 medium yellow onion, chopped
- 1½ cups tomatoes, diced
- 2 tablespoons tomato paste
- 2 tablespoons olive oil
- 2 stalks celery, thinly sliced
- 2 teaspoons dried dill
- 2 teaspoons ground cinnamon
- 2 tablespoons mild paprika
- 2 teaspoons ground cumin
- 1 teaspoon salt
- 1 teaspoon ground black pepper
- 3 cups vegetable broth

Directions:

1. Put the olive oil, celery and onions in the Instant Pot and select "Sauté".
2. Sauté for 4 minutes and add dill, cinnamon, paprika, cumin, salt and black pepper.
3. Sauté for 2 minutes and add chickpeas, beans, tomatoes, lentils and tomato paste.
4. Set the instant pot to "Manual" and cook for 20 minutes at high pressure.
5. Release the pressure naturally and serve hot.

Nutritional Information per Serving:

Calories: 532; Total Fat: 12.6g; Carbs: 79.6g; Sugars: 11.6g; Protein: 30.4g; Cholesterol: 0mg; Sodium: 1198mg

48.Spinach Lentil

Yield: 3 Servings, Prep Time: 10 Minutes, Cook Time: 5 Minutes

Ingredients

- 1 cup spinach, chopped
- ½cup split pigeon pea, washed
- ¼ teaspoon cumin seeds
- 2 garlic cloves, finely chopped
- 1½ cups water
- ½tablespoon oil
- ½ inch ginger, finely chopped
- 1tomato, chopped
- ½teaspoon salt

Directions:

1. Put the oil, garlic, ginger and cumin seeds in the Instant Pot and select "Sauté".
2. Sauté for 35 seconds and add tomato paste and salt.
3. Add the water and lentils and mix well.
4. Set the instant pot to "Manual" and cook for 4 minutes at high pressure.
5. Release the pressure quickly and open the lid.
6. Add spinach and select "Sauté".
7. Sauté for 3 minutes and dish out.

Nutritional Information per Serving:

Calories: 147; Total Fat: 3.1g; Carbs: 23.1g; Sugars: 1.98g; Protein: 8.3g; Cholesterol: 0mg; Sodium: 414mg

49.Confetti Rice

Yield: 4 Servings, Prep Time: 5 Minutes, Cook Time: 12 Minutes

Ingredients

- 1 cup lengthy grain white rice
- 3 cups frozen peas, thawed
- 3 tablespoons butter
- 2 cloves garlic, minced
- 1 cup vegetable broth
- ¼ cup lemon juice
- 1 small onion, chopped
- 1 tablespoon cumin powder
- ½ teaspoon salt
- ½ teaspoon black pepper

Directions:

1. Put the butter and onions in the Instant Pot and select "Sauté".
2. Sauté for 3 minutes and add rest of the ingredients.
3. Set the instant pot to "Manual" and cook for 8 minutes at high pressure.
4. Release the pressure naturally and serve with some freshly grated coriander leaves.

Nutritional Information per Serving:

Calories: 333; Total Fat: 13.5g; Carbs: 40.6g; Sugars: 9.4g; Protein: 13.2g; Cholesterol: 31mg; Sodium: 627mg

50.Coconut Rice

Yield: 4 Servings, Prep Time: 5 Minutes, Cook Time: 10 Minutes

Ingredients

- 1 cup unsweetened coconut, scraped or grated
- 1½ cup lengthy grain white rice
- 3 tablespoons butter
- 3 cups water
- ½ cup currants
- 1 teaspoon cinnamon powder
- ¼ teaspoon cloves
- ¾ teaspoon salt

Directions:

1. Put the butter and all the ingredients except rice and water in the Instant Pot and select "Sauté".
2. Sauté for 2 minutes and add rice and water.
3. Set the instant pot to "Manual" and cook for 6 minutes at high pressure.
4. Release the pressure naturally and dish out.

Nutritional Information per Serving:

Calories: 353; Total Fat: 26.9g; Carbs: 26.8g; Sugars: 3.1g; Protein: 3.7g; Cholesterol: 23mg; Sodium: 515mg

51.Bok Choy Rice

Yield: 5 Servings, Prep Time: 10 Minutes, Cook Time: 12 Minutes

Ingredients

- 1½ cups rice
- 3 cups chopped bokchoy, leaves and stems trimmed
- 1 tablespoon olive oil
- ½ cup garlic, chopped
- ½ cup onions, chopped
- 3 cups hot vegetable broth
- ½ cup white wine
- ½ teaspoon red pepper flakes
- ½ teaspoon salt

Directions:

1. Put the olive oil, onions and garlic in the Instant Pot and select "Sauté".
2. Sauté for 4 minutes and add rice, vegetable broth and wine.
3. Set the instant pot to "Manual" and cook for 6 minutes at high pressure.
4. Release the pressure naturally and add bokchoy.
5. Let it simmer for 5 minutes.

Nutritional Information per Serving:

Calories: 286; Total Fat: 3.4g; Carbs: 53.4g; Sugars: 2.6g; Protein: 5.6g; Cholesterol: 0mg; Sodium: 585mg

52.Sunny Lentils

Yield: 4 Servings, Prep Time: 10 Minutes, Cook Time: 15 Minutes

Ingredients

- 1 cup red lentils
- 1 tablespoon olive oil
- 1/3 cup green bell pepper, chopped
- 1 tablespoon garlic, minced
- 1/3 cup onions, chopped
- 1/3 cup red bell pepper, chopped
- ½ teaspoon dried tarragon
- 1 cup tomatoes, diced
- 3 tablespoons sweetened coconut, shredded
- ¼ teaspoon curry powder
- ½ cup water
- Salt and black pepper, to taste

Directions:

1. Put the olive oil, onions, garlic, green bell pepper, red bell pepper, tarragon and spices in the Instant Pot and select "Sauté".
2. Sauté for 5 minutes and add tomatoes, red lentils and coconut.
3. Set the instant pot to "Manual" and cook for 8 minutes at high pressure.
4. Release the pressure naturally and dish out..

Nutritional Information per Serving:

Calories: 235; Total Fat: 5.5g; Carbs: 34.4g; Sugars: 3.8g; Protein: 13.4g; Cholesterol: 0mg; Sodium: 8mg

53.Coconut Red Lentil Curry

Yield: 6 Servings, Prep Time: 5 Minutes, Cook Time: 30 Minutes

Ingredients

- 1 cup red kidney beans, soaked overnight
- 1½ cups black gram beans, soaked overnight
- 2 cups coconut cream
- 2 cups water
- 2 tablespoons oil
- 2 teaspoons cumin seeds
- 1 cup onions, finely diced
- ½ teaspoon turmeric powder
- 3 tablespoons fresh ginger, grated
- 3 cups tomatoes, diced
- ½ cup cilantro
- 3 teaspoons salt
- 3 teaspoons red chilli powder
- 2 teaspoons garam masala

Directions:

1. Put the oil, onions and cumin seeds in the Instant Pot and select "Sauté".
2. Sauté for 4 minutes and add tomatoes, turmeric powder, ginger, salt, red chilli powder and beans.
3. Sauté for 3 minutes and add water.
4. Set the instant pot to "Manual" mode for 18 minutes at high pressure.
5. Release the pressure naturally for 5 minutes and stir in coconut cream and garam masala.

Nutritional Information per Serving:

Calories: 422; Total Fat: 24.7g; Carbs: 41.3g; Sugars: 6.6g; Protein: 14g; Cholesterol: 0mg; Sodium: 1190mg

54.Creamy Mushroom Alfredo Rice

Yield: 4 Servings, Prep Time: 5 Minutes, Cook Time: 10 Minutes

Ingredients

- 1 cup rice
- 2 tablespoons olive oil
- 2¾ cups vegetable stock
- ¾ cup onions, finely chopped
- 2 garlic cloves, minced
- 1½ tablespoons fresh lemon juice
- 2 oz. Bertolli creamy mushroom Alfredo sauce
- Salt and black pepper, to taste
- ¼ cup walnuts, coarsely chopped

Directions:

1. Put the olive oil, onions and garlic in the Instant Pot and select "Sauté".
2. Sauté for 3 minutes and add rice and vegetable broth.
3. Set the instant pot to "Manual" mode for 5 minutes at high pressure.
4. Release the pressure naturally and add lemon juice, salt, black pepper and Bertolli creamy mushroom Alfredo sauce.
5. Garnish with chopped walnuts and serve warm.

Nutritional Information per Serving:

Calories: 332; Total Fat: 15.4g; Carbs: 42.1g; Sugars: 2.3g; Protein: 7g; Cholesterol: 11; Sodium: 117 mg

INNOVATIVE EGG RECIPES

55.Zesty Eggs

Yield: 4 Servings, Prep Time: 10 Minutes, Cook Time: 8 Minutes

Ingredients

- 4 eggs
- 1½ tablespoons Greek yogurt
- 1½ tablespoons mayonnaise
- 1 teaspoon jalapeno mustard
- ¼ teaspoon onion powder
- ¼ teaspoon paprika
- ¼ teaspoon lemon zests
- Salt and black pepper, to taste

Directions:

1. Place the trivet inside the Instant Pot and add eggs and water.
2. Set the instant pot to "Manual" mode for 6 minutes at high pressure.
3. Release the pressure naturally and transfer the eggs into ice cold water.
4. Scoop out the egg yolks and mix with rest of the ingredients.
5. Fill the hollow eggs with this mixture and serve.

Nutritional Information per Serving:

Calories: 88; Total Fat: 6.3g; Carbs: 2g; Sugars: 0.8g; Protein: 5.8g; Cholesterol: 165mg; Sodium: 123mg

56.Egg Custard

Yield: 8 Servings, Prep Time: 10 Minutes, Cook Time: 35 Minutes

Ingredients

- 6 eggs
- 24-ounce milk
- ½ cup honey
- ¼ teaspoon ground cinnamon
- ¼ teaspoon ground cardamom
- 1/8 teaspoon ground allspice
- ¼ teaspoon ground ginger
- ¼ teaspoon ground nutmeg
- 1/8 teaspoon ground cloves
- Salt, to taste

Directions:

1. Whisk eggs with all other ingredients and divide evenly into 8 small ramekins.
2. Place the trivet inside the Instant Pot and arrange ramekins in it.
3. Set the instant pot to "Manual" mode for 30 minutes at low pressure.
4. Release the pressure naturally and keep aside to cool.

Nutritional Information per Serving:

Calories: 155; Total Fat: 5.1g; Carbs: 22.1g; Sugars: 21.5g; Protein: 7g; Cholesterol: 130mg; Sodium: 87mg

57.Egg Zucchini

Yield: 2 Servings, Prep Time: 10 Minutes, Cook Time: 5 Minutes

Ingredients

- 1 zucchini, cut into ½ inch round slices
- ½ teaspoon dried dill
- ½ teaspoon paprika
- 1 egg
- 1 tablespoon coconut oil
- 1½ tablespoons coconut flour
- 1 tablespoon milk
- Salt and black pepper, to taste

Directions:

1.Whisk egg and almond milk together in a small bowl.

2.Mix the salt, black pepper, paprika, dried dill and coconut flour in another bowl.

3.Dip the zucchini slices in the egg mixture and then in the dry mixture.

4.Put the coconut oil in the Instant Pot and add the zucchini slices.

5.Set the instant pot to "Manual" mode for 4 minutes at high pressure.

6.Release the pressure naturally and dish out.

Nutritional Information per Serving:

Calories: 134; Total Fat: 10g; Carbs: 8g; Sugars: 2.3g; Protein: 5.1g; Cholesterol: 82mg; Sodium: 45mg

58.Egg and Scallion Omelette

Yield: 2 Servings, Prep Time: 10 Minutes, Cook Time: 5 Minutes

Ingredients

- 2 eggs
- 2 small scallions, chopped
- ¼ teaspoon garlic powder
- ¼ teaspoon sesame seeds
- ½ cup water
- Salt and black pepper, to taste

Directions:

1. Place the trivet in the bottom of Instant Pot and add water.
2. Beat together water, garlic powder, salt and black pepper with eggs.
3. Stir in the scallion and sesame seeds.
4. Transfer the bowl on the trivet.
5. Set the instant pot to "Manual" mode for 5 minutes at high pressure.
6. Release the pressure quickly and dish out.

Nutritional Information per Serving:

Calories: 68; Total Fat: 4.6g; Carbs: 1.1g; Sugars: 0.6g; Protein: 5.8g; Cholesterol: 164mg; Sodium: 64mg

59.Egg Veggie Pie

Yield: 8 Servings, Prep Time: 10 Minutes, Cook Time: 10 Minutes

Ingredients

- 16 eggs, beaten
- 2 sweet potatoes, peeled and shredded
- 2 red bell peppers, seeded and chopped
- 2 onions, chopped
- 2 garlic cloves, minced
- 4 teaspoons fresh basil, chopped
- Salt and black pepper, to taste

Directions:

1. Put all the ingredients in the Instant Pot and mix well.
2. Set the instant pot to "Manual" and cook for 8 minutes at high pressure.
3. Release the pressure naturally and dish out.

Nutritional Information per Serving:

Calories: 192; Total Fat: 8.9g; Carbs: 16.2g; Sugars: 3.6g; Protein: 12.3g; Cholesterol: 327mg; Sodium: 129mg

60.Quick Scrambled Eggs

Yield: 1 Serving, Prep Time: 10 Minutes, Cook Time: 5 Minutes

Ingredients

- 2 eggs
- 1 tablespoon milk
- 1 tablespoon butter
- 1 cup water.
- Salt and black pepper, to taste

Directions:

1. Break the eggs in the bowl and add milk, salt and black pepper.
2. Beat gently and add the butter
3. Put water in the Instant pot and arrange the trivet.
4. Put the bowl on the trivet and close the lid.
5. Set the instant pot to "Manual" and cook for 6 minutes at low pressure.
6. Release the pressure quickly and serve hot.

Nutritional Information per Serving:

Calories: 235; Total Fat: 20.6g; Carbs: 1.4g; Sugars: 1.4g; Protein: 11.7g; Cholesterol: 359mg; Sodium: 219mg

61.Turmeric Egg Potatoes

Yield: 3 Servings, Prep Time: 10 Minutes, Cook Time: 10 Minutes

Ingredients

- 2 eggs, whisked
- 1 teaspoon ground turmeric
- 1 teaspoon cumin seeds
- 2 tablespoons olive oil
- 2 potatoes, peeled and diced
- 1 onion, finely chopped
- 2 teaspoons ginger-garlic paste
- ½ teaspoon red chilli powder
- Salt and black pepper, to taste

Directions:

1. Put the olive oil, cumin seeds, ginger-garlic paste and onions in the Instant Pot and select "Sauté".
2. Sauté for 4 minutes and add potatoes and rest of the ingredients.
3. Set the instant pot to "Manual" and cook for 6 minutes at high pressure.
4. Release the pressure naturally and serve warm.

Nutritional Information per Serving:

Calories: 265; Total Fat: 14.7g; Carbs: 28.1g; Sugars: 3.5g; Protein: 6.9g; Cholesterol: 109mg; Sodium: 53mg

62.Egg and Garlic Skillet

Yield: 2 Servings, Prep Time: 5 Minutes, Cook Time: 8 Minutes

Ingredients

- 2 eggs, whisked
- 1 tablespoon olive oil
- 2 tomatoes, cut into 4 halves
- 2 teaspoons garlic, minced
- 1 green onion, chopped
- Salt and black pepper, to taste

Directions:

1. Put the olive oil, garlic and green onions in the Instant Pot and select "Sauté".
2. Sauté for 4 minutes and add tomatoes and eggs.
3. Set the instant pot to "Manual" and cook for 3 minutes at high pressure.
4. Release the pressure naturally and serve warm.

Nutritional Information per Serving:

Calories: 152; Total Fat: 11.6g; Carbs: 6.6g; Sugars: 3.8g; Protein: 6.9g; Cholesterol: 164mg; Sodium: 69mg

63.Egg Pancakes

Yield: 5 Servings, Prep Time: 10 Minutes, Cook Time: 25 Minutes

Ingredients

- 3 eggs
- 2 tablespoons honey
- ½ teaspoon ginger powder
- ½ cup milk
- 4 tablespoons lemon curd
- 1 cup self-rising flour
- 1 tablespoon baking powder
- 1 tablespoon butter, melted
- 3 mango slices

Directions:

1. Mix together self-rising flour, baking powder and ginger powder in a bowl.
2. Put the eggs, milk, honey and butter in it and mix well.
3. Put 2 tablespoons in the baking dish.
4. Place the trivet in the Instant Pot and put the baking dish in it.
5. Set the instant pot to "Manual" and cook for 5 minutes at low pressure.
6. Release the pressure naturally and repeat the process with the remaining mixture.
7. Stack all the pancakes into a plate and top with lemon curd and mango slices.

Nutritional Information per Serving:

Calories: 242; Total Fat: 10.5g; Carbs: 33g; Sugars: 12.3g; Protein: 7.6g; Cholesterol: 146mg; Sodium: 108mg

TASTY SNACKS RECIPES

64. Instant Pot Sauté Nuts

Yield: 6 Servings, Prep Time: 10 Minutes, Cook Time: 20 Minutes

Ingredients

- 1 cup cashews
- 1 cup almonds
- 1 cup pecans
- 1 cup raisins
- 1 tablespoon butter
- ½ teaspoon brown sugar
- ½ teaspoon black pepper
- 1½ teaspoon chilli powder
- ½ teaspoon sea salt
- ½ teaspoon garlic powder
- ¼ teaspoon cayenne pepper
- ½ teaspoon cumin powder

Directions:

1. Put the butter, almonds, cashews, raisins and pecans in the Instant Pot.
2. Season with all the spices and stir gently.
3. Set the instant pot to "Manual" and cook for 20 minutes at high pressure.
4. Release the pressure naturally and serve.

Nutritional Information per Serving:

Calories: 335; Total Fat: 22.4g; Carbs: 31.5g; Sugars: 16.5g; Protein: 8.1g; Cholesterol: 5mg; Sodium: 177mg

65.Mushroom Spinach Treat

Yield: 3 Servings, Prep Time: 10 Minutes, Cook Time: 12 Minutes

Ingredients

- ½ cup spinach
- ½ pound fresh mushrooms, sliced
- 2 garlic cloves, minced
- 2 tablespoons fresh thyme, chopped
- 1 onion, chopped
- 1 tablespoon olive oil
- 1 tablespoon fresh cilantro, chopped
- Salt and black pepper, to taste

Directions:

1. Put the olive oil, garlic and onions in the Instant Pot and select "Sauté".
2. Sauté for 4 minutes and add spinach, mushrooms, salt, black pepper and thyme.
3. Set the instant pot to "Manual" and cook for 7 minutes at high pressure.
4. Release the pressure naturally and garnish with cilantro.

Nutritional Information per Serving:

Calories: 86; Total Fat: 5.32g; Carbs: 8.1g; Sugars: 3g; Protein: 4g; Cholesterol: 0mg; Sodium: 138mg

66.Spicy Roasted Olives

Yield: 4 Servings, Prep Time: 10 Minutes, Cook Time: 7 Minutes

Ingredients

- 2 cups green and black olives, mixed
- 2 tangerines
- 2 garlic cloves, minced
- 2 tablespoons vinegar
- ½ inch piece of turmeric, finely grated
- 1 fresh red chilli, thinly sliced
- 2 sprigs rosemary
- 1 tablespoon olive oil

Directions:

1.Put all the ingredients except the tangerines in the Instant Pot.

2.Squeeze the tangerines in the Instant Pot over all the ingredients.

3.Set the instant pot to "Manual" and cook for 6 minutes at high pressure.

4.Release the pressure naturally and dish out.

Nutritional Information per Serving:

Calories: 163; Total Fat: 13.6g; Carbs: 2.3g; Sugars: 0.5g; Protein: 0.4g; Cholesterol: 0mg; Sodium: 561mg

67.Cooked Guacamole

Yield: 4 Servings, Prep Time: 10 Minutes, Cook Time: 10 Minutes

Ingredients

- 1 large onion, finely diced
- 4 tablespoons lemon juice
- ¼ cup cilantro, chopped
- 4 avocados, peeled and diced
- 3 tablespoons olive oil
- 3 jalapenos, finely diced
- Salt and black pepper, to taste

Directions:

1. Put the olive oil and onions in the Instant Pot and select "Sauté".
2. Sauté for 3 minutes and add cilantro, lemon juice, avocados, salt, black pepper and jalapenos.
3. Set the instant pot to "Manual" and cook for 6 minutes at high pressure.
4. Release the pressure naturally and dish out.

Nutritional Information per Serving:

Calories: 401; Total Fat: 37.4g; Carbs: 19.4g; Sugars: 2.8g; Protein: 4.18g; Cholesterol: 0mg; Sodium: 19mg

68.Butternut Squash

Yield: 2 Servings, Prep Time: 10 Minutes, Cook Time: 7 Minutes

Ingredients

- 1 whole butternut squash, washed
- 1 tablespoon butter
- 1 tablespoon BBQ sauce
- Salt and black pepper, to taste
- ¼ teaspoon smoked paprika

Directions:

1. Season the butternut squash with paprika, salt and pepper.
2. Put the butter and seasoned whole butternut squash in the Instant Pot.
3. Set the instant pot to "Manual" and cook for 6 minutes at high pressure.
4. Release the pressure naturally and top with BBQ sauce.

Nutritional Information per Serving:

Calories: 154; Total Fat: 6.6g; Carbs: 19.5g; Sugars: 5.6g; Protein: 3.1g; Cholesterol: 15mg; Sodium: 318mg

69.Baked Potato

Yield: 2 Servings, Prep Time: 10 Minutes, Cook Time: 30 Minutes

Ingredients

- 2 medium potatoes, well-scrubbed
- 1 tablespoon olive oil
- 2 sheets aluminium foil
- ¼ cup sour cream
- Salt, to taste

Directions:

1. Arrange the trivet in the Instant Pot.
2. Rub the potatoes with olive oil and salt.
3. Wrap the potatoes tightly in the aluminium foil.
4. Transfer the potatoes on the trivet.
5. Set the instant pot to "Manual" and cook for 30 minutes at low pressure.
6. Release the pressure naturally and fill in the sour cream.

Nutritional Information per Serving:

Calories: 269; Total Fat: 13.2g; Carbs: 34.7g; Sugars: 2.5g; Protein: 4.5g; Cholesterol: 13mg; Sodium: 28mg

70.Cajun Spiced Pecans

Yield: 3 Servings, Prep Time: 10 Minutes, Cook Time: 20 Minutes

Ingredients

- ½ pound pecan halves
- 1 teaspoon dried basil
- 1 teaspoon dried thyme
- ½ tablespoon chilli powder
- ¼ teaspoon garlic powder
- ¼ teaspoon cayenne pepper
- 1 tablespoon olive oil
- 1 teaspoon dried oregano
- Salt, to taste

Directions:

1.Put all the ingredients in the Instant Pot.

2.Set the instant pot to "Manual" and cook for 20 minutes at low pressure.

3.Release the pressure naturally and serve.

Nutritional Information per Serving:

Calories: 345; Total Fat: 33.1g; Carbs: 7.2g; Sugars: 0.1g; Protein: 4.4g; Cholesterol: 0mg; Sodium: 0mg

71.Energy Booster Cookies

Yield: 6 Servings, Prep Time: 10 Minutes, Cook Time: 10 Minutes

Ingredients

- 2 large eggs
- 2/3 cup cocoa powder
- 1/3 cup sugar
- 1¼ cups almond butter
- Salt, to taste

Directions:

1. Put all the ingredients in a food processor and pulse.
2. Roll the mixture into 12 equal small balls and press them.
3. Arrange the balls onto a cookie sheet in a single layer.
4. Place the trivet in the Instant Pot and transfer the cookie sheet on it.
5. Set the instant pot to "Manual" and cook for 10 minutes at high pressure.
6. Release the pressure naturally and dish out the cookies.

Nutritional Information per Serving:

Calories: 107; Total Fat: 4.8g; Carbs: 17.1g; Sugars: 11.6g; Protein: 4.5g; Cholesterol: 62mg; Sodium: 25mg

72.Grilled Peaches

Yield: 5 Servings, Prep Time: 7 Minutes, Cook Time: 8 Minutes

Ingredients

- 5 medium peaches
- ¼ teaspoon ground cloves
- ½ teaspoon ground cinnamon
- ½ teaspoon brown sugar
- 2 tablespoons olive oil
- ¼ teaspoon salt

Directions

1. Remove the pits from the peaches and add olive oil on the cut side of the peaches.
2. Sprinkle the peaches with salt, cloves, cinnamon and brown sugar.
3. Place the trivet in the Instant Pot and transfer the peaches on it.
4. Set the instant pot to "Manual" and cook for 7 minutes at high pressure.
5. Release the pressure naturally and dish out.

Nutritional Information per Serving:

Calories: 109; Total Fat: 6g; Carbs: 14.6g; Sugars: 14.3g; Protein: 1.4g; Cholesterol: 0mg; Sodium: 0mg

73.Honey Citrus Roasted Cashews

Yield: 2 Servings, Prep Time: 10 Minutes, Cook Time: 25 Minutes

Ingredients

- ¾ cup cashews
- ¼ teaspoon salt
- ¼ teaspoon ginger powder
- 1 teaspoon orange zest, minced
- 4 tablespoons honey

Directions

1. Mix together honey, orange zest, ginger powder and salt.
2. Add cashews to this mixture and place it in a ramekin.
3. Place the trivet in the Instant Pot and transfer the cashews on it.
4. Set the instant pot to "Manual" and cook for 20 minutes at high pressure.
5. Release the pressure naturally and dish out.

Nutritional Information per Serving:

Calories: 292; Total Fat: 12.3g; Carbs: 43g; Sugars: 34.5g; Protein: 5.2g; Cholesterol: 0mg; Sodium: 295mg

74.Pumpkin Muffins

Yield: 10 Servings, Prep Time: 10 Minutes, Cook Time: 15 Minutes

Ingredients

- 2 cups almond flour
- 4 tablespoons coconut flour
- 1½ teaspoons baking soda
- 2 teaspoons pumpkin pie spice
- ¼ teaspoon salt
- 1 cup pumpkin puree
- 3 teaspoons almond butter
- 1½ teaspoons baking powder
- ½ teaspoon ground cinnamon
- 3 large eggs
- ½ cup raw honey
- 2 tablespoon almonds, toasted and chopped

Directions:

1. Whisk together almond flour, coconut flour, cinnamon, baking soda, baking powder, salt and pumpkin pie spice.
2. Whisk together eggs, honey, pumpkin puree and butter.
3. Combine both the wet and dry mixtures.
4. Fill inside the muffin cups and top with almonds.
5. Place the trivet in the Instant Pot and transfer the muffin cups on it.
6. Set the instant pot to "Manual" and cook for 12 minutes at high pressure.
7. Release the pressure naturally and dish out.

Nutritional Information per Serving:

Calories: 268; Total Fat: 15.9g; Carbs: 25.7g; Sugars: 15.1g; Protein: 8.7g; Cholesterol: 56mg; Sodium: 784mg

75.Banana Chips

Yield: 3 Servings, Prep Time: 10 Minutes, Cook Time: 30 Minutes

Ingredients

- 3 bananas, cut into 1/8 inch slices
- 3 tablespoons lemon juice
- 3 tablespoons nutmeg

Directions

1. Mix together all the ingredients in a bowl.
2. Spread banana slices evenly over baking sheet in one layer.
3. Place the trivet in the Instant Pot and transfer the baking sheet on it.
4. Set the instant pot to "Manual" and cook for 25 minutes at high pressure.
5. Release the pressure naturally and dish out.

Nutritional Information per Serving:

Calories: 145; Total Fat: 3.1g; Carbs: 30.7g; Sugars: 16.7g; Protein: 1.8g; Cholesterol: 0mg; Sodium: 5mg

76.Mustard Flavoured Artichokes

Yield: 3 Servings, Prep Time: 10 Minutes, Cook Time: 15 Minutes

Ingredients

- 3 artichokes
- 3 tablespoons mayonnaise
- 1 cup water
- 2 pinches paprika
- 2 lemons, sliced in half
- 2 teaspoons Dijon mustard

Directions:

1. Mix together mayonnaise, paprika and Dijon mustard.
2. Place the trivet in the Instant Pot and add water.
3. Put the artichokes upwards and arrange lemon slices on it.
4. Set the instant pot to "Manual" and cook for 12 minutes at high pressure.
5. Release the pressure naturally and put the artichokes in the mayonnaise mixture.

Nutritional Information per Serving:

Calories: 147; Total Fat: 5.4g; Carbs: 24.4g; Sugars: 3.6g; Protein: 6g; Cholesterol: 4mg; Sodium: 298mg

SCRUMPTIOUS DESSERT RECIPES

77.Sweet Potato Dessert Risotto

Yield: 6 Servings, Prep Time: 10 Minutes, Cook Time: 18 Minutes

Ingredients

- ½ cup risotto rice
- ½ cup coconut milk
- 1 tablespoon butter
- ¾ cup water
- ½ teaspoon vanilla extract
- ½ teaspoon cardamom powder
- ½ cup raisins
- ½ cup evaporated milk
- ¼ cup honey
- ½ teaspoon cinnamon powder
- ½ teaspoon salt
- 1 sweet potato, grated
- ½ cup almonds, roasted and grated

Directions:

1. Put the butter and melt it in the Instant Pot.
2. Add evaporated milk, coconut milk, honey and water.
3. Mix well and add cardamom powder, cinnamon powder, vanilla extract and salt.
4. Stir well and add risotto rice and grated sweet potato.
5. Set the Instant Pot to "Manual" at high pressure for 12 minutes.
6. Release the pressure naturally and add raisins.
7. Let it simmer for 4 minutes and top with roasted almonds.

Nutritional Information per Serving:

Calories: 291; Total Fat: 12.4g; Carbs: 42.5g; Sugars: 23.2g; Protein: 5.5g; Cholesterol: 11mg; Sodium: 243mg

78.Sweet Caramel Coffee

Yield: 3 Servings, Prep Time: 10 Minutes, Cook Time: 20 Minutes

Ingredients

- 4 egg yolks
- 1 cup heavy cream
- ½ teaspoon coffee powder
- Pinch of salt
- ¼ cup granulated sugar
- ½ teaspoon vanilla extract
- 3 tablespoons superfine sugar
- 1 cup water

Directions:

1. Whisk egg yolks, granulated sugar and salt in a bowl.
2. Add coffee powder, heavy cream and vanilla extract and whisk gently.
3. Put this mixture in 3 custard cups and cover tightly with an aluminium foil.
4. Arrange the trivet in the Instant Pot and add water.
5. Place the custard cups on the trivet and lock the lid.
6. Set the instant pot to "Manual" and cook for 6 minutes at high pressure.
7. Release the pressure naturally for 10 minutes and remove the cups.
8. Refrigerate the caramel and sprinkle superfine sugar.
9. Burn this sprinkled sugar for 2 minutes using a blow torch.

Nutritional Information per Serving:

Calories: 337; Total Fat: 20.8g; Carbs: 35.4g; Sugars: 33.6g; Protein: 4.4g; Cholesterol: 335mg; Sodium: 79mg

79.Red Wine Poached Pears

Yield: 3 Servings, Prep Time: 10 Minutes, Cook Time: 30 Minutes

Ingredients

- 3 firm pears, peeled and stem attached
- ½ bottle red wine
- 2 cloves
- ½ teaspoon ginger, grated
- ½ cinnamon, grated
- 1 bay laurel leaf
- 1 cup granulated sugar

Directions:

1. Put all the ingredients in the Instant Pot and lock the lid.
2. Set the instant pot to "Manual" and cook for 8 minutes at high pressure.
3. Release the pressure naturally for 10 minutes and dish out the pears.
4. Let the mixture simmer for 10 more minutes to reduce its consistency.
5. Drizzle the red wine sauce on pears and serve.

Nutritional Information per Serving:

Calories: 434; Total Fat: 0.38g; Carbs: 101.7g; Sugars: 87.9g; Protein: 1.2g; Cholesterol: 0mg; Sodium: 6mg

80.Cherry Apple Risotto

Yield: 4 Servings, Prep Time: 10 Minutes, Cook Time: 10 Minutes

Ingredients

- 1 tablespoon butter
- ¾ cup Arborio rice, soaked
- 1 apple, diced
- 2 pinches salt
- ¾ teaspoon cinnamon powder
- ¼ cup brown sugar
- ½ cup apple juice
- 1½ cups milk
- ¼ cup dried cherries
- 1½ tablespoons almonds, roasted and sliced
- ¼ cup whipped cream

Directions:

1. Put the butter and rice in the Instant Pot and select "Sauté".
2. Sauté for 3 minutes and add rest of the ingredients.
3. Set the Instant Pot to "Manual" at high pressure for 7 minutes.
4. Release the pressure quickly and add dried cherries, almonds and whipped cream.

Nutritional Information per Serving:

Calories: 317; Total Fat: 8.5g; Carbs: 54.9g; Sugars: 21.8g; Protein: 6.2g; Cholesterol: 23mg; Sodium: 151mg

81.Coconut Chocolate Fondue

Yield: 4 Servings, Prep Time: 10 Minutes, Cook Time: 5 Minutes

Ingredients

- 1 cup Swiss bittersweet chocolate (70%)
- 1 cup coconut cream
- 2teaspoons coconut milk powder
- 2 teaspoons sugar
- 2 teaspoons coconut essence
- 2 cups water

Directions:

1. Mix chocolate, sugar and coconut cream in a ceramic pot.
2. Arrange the trivet in the Instant Pot and add water.
3. Place the ceramic pot on the trivet and lock the lid.
4. Set the instant pot to "Manual" and cook for 3 minutes at high pressure.
5. Release the pressure naturally and add coconut essence and coconut milk powder.
6. Stir gently and serve in fondue pot.

Nutritional Information per Serving:

Calories: 266; Total Fat: 21.4g; Carbs: 16.8g; Sugars: 14.2g; Protein: 2.7g; Cholesterol: 0mg; Sodium: 26mg

82.Strawberry Rhubarb Tarts

Yield: 12 Servings, Prep Time: 10 Minutes, Cook Time: 7 Minutes

Ingredients

- 1 cup water
- 1 pound rhubarb, cut into ½ inch pieces
- ½ pound strawberries
- ¼ cup crystallized ginger, chopped
- Readymade 12 tart shells, short crust
- ½ cup honey
- ½ cup whipped cream

Directions:

1. Put all the ingredients in the Instant Pot except the tart shells and whipped cream.
2. Set the instant pot to "Manual" and cook for 5 minutes at high pressure.
3. Release the pressure naturally and fill the mixture in the tart shells.
4. Top with whipped cream and serve.

Nutritional Information per Serving:

Calories: 163; Total Fat: 6.2g; Carbs: 26.2g; Sugars: 14g; Protein: 1.6g; Cholesterol: 11mg; Sodium: 90mg

83. Sweet Milk

Yield: 2 Servings, Prep Time: 10 Minutes, Cook Time: 45 Minutes

Ingredients

- 2 cans(14 oz.) sweetened condensed milk
- 16 cups water
- 2 (16 oz.) canning jar with lid

Directions:

1. Pour condensed milk in the canning jar, place the lid and screw on the ring.
2. Arrange the trivet in the Instant Pot and add water.
3. Place the canning jar on the trivet and lock the lid.
4. Set the instant pot to "Manual" and cook for 30 minutes at high pressure.
5. Release the pressure naturally for 15 minutes and let it cool.

Nutritional Information per Serving:

Calories: 61; Total Fat: 1.7g; Carbs: 10.4g; Sugars: 10.4g; Protein: 1.5g; Cholesterol: 6mg; Sodium: 81mg

84.Hazelnut Flan

Yield: 10 Servings, Prep Time: 10 Minutes, Cook Time: 10 Minutes

Ingredients

- 6 eggs
- ½ cups granulated sugar
- 4 cups whole milk
- 2 teaspoons vanilla extract
- 4 egg yolks
- ¼ teaspoon salt
- 1 cup whipping cream
- 8 tablespoons hazelnut syrup
- ½ cup caramel
- 2 cups water

Directions:

1. Whisk together eggs, egg yolks, salt and sugar in a bowl.
2. Boil milk and add gradually to the egg mixture.
3. Add vanilla extract, whipping cream and hazelnut syrup to this mixture.
4. Put the caramel in the custard cups and add the hazelnut mixture in them.
5. Arrange the trivet in the Instant Pot and add water.
6. Place the custard cups on the trivet and lock the lid.
7. Set the instant pot to "Manual" and cook for 8 minutes at high pressure.
8. Release the pressure naturally and serve after refrigerating it for 3 hours.

Nutritional Information per Serving:

Calories: 244; Total Fat: 14.2g; Carbs: 21.4g; Sugars: 20.32g; Protein: 8.5g; Cholesterol: 206mg; Sodium: 160mg

85.Peanut Butter Custard

Yield: 10 Servings, Prep Time: 10 Minutes, Cook Time: 10 Minutes

Ingredients

- 1 cup caramel
- 4 whole eggs
- 4 egg yolks
- ½ cup granulated sugar
- ¼ teaspoon salt
- 4 cups whole milk
- 1 cup whipping cream
- 2 teaspoons vanilla extract
- 8 tablespoons peanut butter
- 2 cups water

Directions:

1. Whisk together eggs, egg yolks, salt and sugar in a bowl.
2. Boil milk and add gradually to the egg mixture.
3. Add vanilla extract, whipping cream and peanut butter to this mixture.
4. Put the caramel in the custard cups and add the peanut butter mixture in them.
5. Arrange the trivet in the Instant Pot and add water.
6. Place the custard cups on the trivet and lock the lid.
7. Set the instant pot to "Manual" and cook for 10 minutes at high pressure.
8. Release the pressure naturally and serve after refrigerating it for 3 hours.

Nutritional Information per Serving:

Calories: 276; Total Fat: 17.3g; Carbs: 21.9g; Sugars: 20.1g; Protein: 10.1g;

Cholesterol: 173mg; Sodium: 203mg

86.Cranberry Apple Rice Pudding

Yield: 4 Servings, Prep Time: 10 Minutes, Cook Time: 10 Minutes

Ingredients

- ¾ cup Arborio rice, soaked
- 2 pinches salt
- ¼ cup brown sugar
- 1½ cups milk
- 1½ tablespoons almonds, roasted and sliced
- 1 tablespoon butter
- 1 apple, diced
- ¾ teaspoon cinnamon powder
- ½ cup apple juice
- ¼ cup dried cranberries
- ¼ cup whipped cream

Directions:

1. Put the butter and rice in the Instant Pot and select "Sauté".
2. Sauté for 4 minutes and add rest of the ingredients.
3. Set the Instant Pot to "Manual" at high pressure for 8 minutes.
4. Release the pressure quickly and add dried cranberries, almonds and whipped cream.

Nutritional Information per Serving:

Calories: 317; Total Fat: 8.5g; Carbs: 5.9g; Sugars: 21.8g; Protein: 6.2g; Cholesterol: 23mg; Sodium: 151mg

87.Chocolate Pudding

Yield: 6 Servings, Prep Time: 10 Minutes, Cook Time: 23 Minutes

Ingredients

- 2 tablespoons dark chocolate, grated
- 1/2 cup golden castor sugar
- 1 teaspoon vanilla extract
- 1 tablespoon cocoa powder
- 1/2 cup butter
- 2 eggs
- 1/2 cup self-rising flour
- 2 cups water

Directions:

1. Mix together butter, sugar, eggs and vanilla extract in a bowl.
2. Sift self-rising flour, dark chocolate and cocoa powder in the eggs mixture.
3. Arrange the trivet in the Instant Pot and add water.
4. Put the bowl on the trivet and lock the lid.
5. Set the Instant Pot to "Manual" at low pressure for 20 minutes.
6. Release the pressure naturally and refrigerate before serving.

Nutritional Information per Serving:

Calories: 287; Total Fat: 16.3g; Carbs: 31.9g; Sugars: 18.3g; Protein: 4.2g; Cholesterol: 91mg; Sodium: 30mg

88.Dark Chocolate Fondue

Yield: 3 Servings, Prep Time: 10 Minutes, Cook Time: 5 Minutes

Ingredients

- 3/4 cup Swiss bittersweet chocolate (70%)
- 3/4 cup fresh cream
- 1½ teaspoons Amaretto Liquor
- 1½ teaspoons sugar
- 1½ cups water

Directions:

1. Mix chocolate, sugar and fresh cream in a ceramic pot.
2. Arrange the trivet in the Instant Pot and add water.
3. Place the ceramic pot on the trivet and lock the lid.
4. Set the instant pot to "Manual" and cook for 3 minutes at high pressure.
5. Release the pressure naturally and add Amaretto Liquor.
6. Stir gently and serve in fondue pot.

Nutritional Information per Serving:

Calories: 399; Total Fat: 27.4g; Carbs: 38.3g; Sugars: 31g; Protein: 4.1g; Cholesterol: 38mg; Sodium: 86mg

89.White Chocolate Orange Fondue

Yield: 6 Servings, Prep Time: 10 Minutes, Cook Time: 5 Minutes

Ingredients

- 1 cup Swiss white chocolate
- 1 cup fresh cream
- 2½ teaspoons candied orange peel, chopped finely
- 2½ teaspoons sugar
- 2½ teaspoons orange essence
- 2½ cups water

Directions:

1. Mix white chocolate, sugar and fresh cream in a ceramic pot.
2. Arrange the trivet in the Instant Pot and add water.
3. Place the ceramic pot on the trivet and lock the lid.
4. Set the instant pot to "Manual" and cook for 4 minutes at high pressure.
5. Release the pressure naturally and add candied orange peel and orange essence.
6. Stir gently and serve in fondue pot.

Nutritional Information per Serving:

Calories: 379; Total Fat: 22.6g; Carbs: 38g; Sugars: 34.9g; Protein: 3.8g; Cholesterol: 40mg; Sodium: 105mg

90.Instant Pot Baked Apple

Yield: 3 Serving, Prep Time: 3 Minutes, Cook Time: 12 Minutes

Ingredients

- 3 apples, cored
- ¼ cup raisins
- ½ cup red wine
- ¼ cup sugar
- ½ teaspoon cinnamon powder

Directions:

1. Put all the ingredients in the Instant Pot and lock the lid.
2. Set the instant pot to "Manual" and cook for 10 minutes at high pressure.
3. Release the pressure naturally and serve hot.

Nutritional Information per Serving:

Calories: 247; Total Fat: 0.5g; Carbs: 58.1g; Sugars: 47.3g; Protein: 1g; Cholesterol: 0mg; Sodium: 5mg

91.Chocolate Hazelnut Lava Cake

Yield: 4 Servings, Prep Time: 10 Minutes, Cook Time: 10 Minutes

Ingredients

- ½ cup all-purpose flour
- ¼ cup hazelnut paste
- 2 tablespoons fresh cream
- ½ cup sugar
- 1 pinch salt
- 4tablespoons bitter cocoa powder
- ½ teaspoon baking powder
- 1 medium egg
- ¾ cup milk
- ¼ cup olive oil
- 1 cup water

Directions:

1. Mix together flour, sugar, salt, baking powder and cocoa powder in a bowl.
2. Add egg, olive oil, milk and whisk well.
3. Put this mixture into 4 small ramekins and put hazelnut paste in the centre.
4. Arrange the trivet in the Instant Pot and add water.
5. Place the ramekins on the trivet and lock the lid.
6. Set the instant pot to "Manual" and cook for 10 minutes at high pressure.
7. Release the pressure naturally and serve hot.

Nutritional Information per Serving:

Calories: 355; Total Fat: 19.3g; Carbs: 44.4g; Sugars: 28.2g; Protein: 6.4g;

Cholesterol: 46mg; Sodium: 80mg

92.Pear and Apple Clafoutis

Yield: 8 Servings, Prep Time: 10 Minutes, Cook Time: 25 Minutes

Ingredients

- 2 eggs
- 1 cup apples, chopped
- 1 cup pears, chopped
- ¾ cup sugar
- 2 cups all-purpose flour
- 1 cup milk
- 1 tablespoon vanilla extract
- 2 tablespoons powdered sugar
- 2 cups water
- Oil, for greasing

Directions

1. Oil the wax paper and place it well in the tin.
2. Mix together eggs, vanilla extract and sugar in a bowl.
3. Add milk and flour gradually and pour in the tin.
4. Top with chopped fruits and cover tightly with the foil.
5. Arrange the trivet in the Instant Pot and add water.
6. Place the tin on the trivet and lock the lid.
7. Set the instant pot to "Manual" and cook for 20 minutes at high pressure.
8. Release the pressure naturally and serve hot.

Nutritional Information per Serving:

Calories: 254; Total Fat: 2.1g; Carbs: 53.3g; Sugars: 27.3g; Protein: 5.8g; Cholesterol: 43mg; Sodium: 33mg

93.Almond and Cardamom Tapioca Pudding

Yield: 4 Servings, Prep Time: 10 Minutes, Cook Time: 5 Minutes

Ingredients

- 1/4 cup tapioca pearls
- ½ cup water
- ½ teaspoon cardamom powder
- 1 cup whole milk
- ½ cup sugar
- ½ cup almonds, roasted

Directions:

1. Mix together tapioca pearls, milk, sugar, cardamom powder and water in a bowl.
2. Arrange the trivet in the Instant Pot and add 2 cups water.
3. Place the bowl on the trivet and lock the lid.
4. Set the instant pot to "Manual" and cook for 8 minutes at high pressure.
5. Release the pressure naturally and garnish with almonds.

Nutritional Information per Serving:

Calories: 245; Total Fat: 7.9g; Carbs: 41.6g; Sugars: 29.1g; Protein: 4.5g; Cholesterol: 6mg; Sodium: 26mg

Hot and Cold Beverages Recipes

94.Agua De Jamaica Hibiscus Tea

Yield: 8 Servings , Prep Time: 5 Minutes, Cook Time: 15 Minutes

Ingredients

- 1 cup hibiscus flowers, dried
- 2 quarts water
- 1 cup sugar
- ½teaspoon ginger, minced
- 1 cinnamon stick
- 2 teaspoons lime juice

Directions:

1. Put all the ingredients in the Instant Pot except lime juice.
2. Set the instant pot to "Manual" and cook for 5 minutes at high pressure.
3. Release the pressure naturally for 10 minutes and decant the liquid into a glass pitcher.
4. Add lime juice to the pitcher and serve after chilling.

Nutritional Information per Serving:

Calories: 95; Total Fat: 0g; Carbs: 25.4g; Sugars: 25g; Protein: 4g; Cholesterol: 0mg; Sodium: 7mg

95.Blackberry Drink

Yield: 4 Servings, Prep Time: 5 Minutes, Cook Time: 15 Minutes

Ingredients

- 2 cups blackberries
- 1 bottle water
- 1 cup white sugar
- 1 lemon, roundly sliced

Directions:

1. Put all the ingredients in the Instant Pot except lemon.
2. Set the instant pot to "Manual" and cook for 10 minutes at high pressure.
3. Release the pressure naturally and decant the liquid into serving glasses.
4. Add lemon slices to the serving glasses and serve after chilling.

Nutritional Information per Serving:

Calories: 223; Total Fat: 0.4g; Carbs: 58.3g; Sugars: 53.9g; Protein: 1.2g; Cholesterol: 0mg; Sodium: 3mg

96.Spiked Cider

Yield: 3 Servings , Prep Time: 5 Minutes, Cook Time: 15 Minutes

Ingredients

- 3 apples, sliced
- 1 orange, sliced
- ¼ teaspoon nutmeg
- ½ cup fresh cranberries
- 2 cinnamon sticks
- 3 cups water
- 3 tablespoons organic cassava syrup

Directions:

1. Put all the ingredients in the Instant Pot.
2. Set the instant pot to "Manual" and cook for 10 minutes at high pressure.
3. Release the pressure naturally and strain the mixture using mesh strainer.

Nutritional Information per Serving:

Calories: 162; Total Fat: 0.6g; Carbs: 41.7g; Sugars: 29.7g; Protein: 1.3g; Cholesterol: 0mg; Sodium: 9mg

97.Berry Kombucha

Yield: 6 Servings , Prep Time: 2 Minutes, Cook Time: 10 Minutes

Ingredients

- 4 cups sparkling water
- 1 cup frozen mixed berries
- 4 cups kombucha

Directions:

1. Put all the ingredients in the Instant Pot.
2. Set the instant pot to "Manual" and cook for 8 minutes at high pressure.
3. Release the pressure naturally and serve hot.

Nutritional Information per Serving:

Calories: 31; Total Fat: 0.1g; Carbs: 7g; Sugars: 2.9g; Protein: 0.2g; Cholesterol: 0mg; Sodium: 7mg

98.Berry Lemonade Tea

Yield: 4 Servings , Prep Time: 5 Minutes, Cook Time: 15 Minutes

Ingredients

- 3 tea bags
- 2 cups natural lemonade
- 1 cup frozen mixed berries
- 2 cups water
- 1 lemon, sliced

Directions:

1. Put all the ingredients in the Instant Pot.
2. Set the instant pot to "Manual" and cook for 12 minutes at high pressure.
3. Release the pressure naturally and strain the mixture.

Nutritional Information per Serving:

Calories: 8; Total Fat: 0.2g; Carbs: 21.6g; Sugars: 18.4g; Protein: 0.4g; Cholesterol: 0mg; Sodium: 4mg

99.Ginger Lemon Tea

Yield: 4 Servings , Prep Time: 10 Minutes, Cook Time: 17 Minutes

Ingredients

- 3 cups water
- 1 (1-inch) piece fresh ginger, peeled
- 1 cup fresh lemon juice
- 1 teaspoon ginger powder
- 1 tablespoon fenugreek seeds

Directions:

1. Put all the ingredients in the Instant Pot.
2. Set the instant pot to "Manual" and cook for 15 minutes at high pressure.
3. Release the pressure naturally and strain the mixture.

Nutritional Information per Serving:

Calories: 27; Total Fat: 0.7g; Carbs: 3.5g; Sugars: 1.3g; Protein: 1.2g; Cholesterol: 0mg; Sodium: 20mg

100.Spiced Ginger Cider

Yield: 12 Servings, Prep Time: 10 Minutes, Cook Time: 15 Minutes

Ingredients

- 2 small apples, peeled
- 12 cups apple cider
- 2 whole allspice
- 2 teaspoons fresh ginger
- 4 teaspoons orange zest
- 2 teaspoons cinnamon powder
- 4 whole cloves
- ½ teaspoon ground nutmeg

Directions:

1. Put all the ingredients in the Instant Pot.
2. Set the instant pot to "Manual" and cook for 13 minutes at high pressure.
3. Release the pressure naturally and strain the mixture.

Nutritional Information per Serving:

Calories: 141; Total Fat: 0.6g; Carbs: 35.2g; Sugars: 31g; Protein: 0.4g; Cholesterol: 0mg; Sodium: 10mg

101.Swedish Glögg

Yield: 1 Serving, Prep Time: 5 Minutes, Cook Time: 18 Minutes

Ingredients

- ½ cup orange juice
- ½ cup water
- 1 (½-inch) piece fresh ginger
- 1 whole clove
- 1 cardamom pods, opened
- 2 tablespoons orange zest
- 1 cinnamon stick
- 1 whole allspice
- 1 vanilla bean

Directions:

1. Put all the ingredients in the Instant Pot.
2. Set the instant pot to "Manual" and cook for 15 minutes at high pressure.
3. Release the pressure naturally and strain the mixture.

Nutritional Information per Serving:

Calories: 194; Total Fat: 3.1g; Carbs: 41.4g; Sugars: 10.5g; Protein: 1.7g; Cholesterol: 10mg; Sodium: 64mg

RECIPE INDEX

CONCLUSION

If you want to have delicious and healthy vegetarian diet using an instant pot, than this is the solution for your problem. This recipe book not only provides you with 150 vegetarian recipes from almost are food groups, but also the procedure to cook them in an instant pot. Cooking had never been this easy for you than before, so don't waste your time and get a hold of this recipe book.

The recipes in the book are easily to cook and will enable you to become an outstanding chef in a very short time. The Instant Pot will help you out in having these delicious recipes to yourself in a less time, without much effort and yet the food you will serve yourself and your loved ones will have no match to it whether it is the taste or the nutrients, it can never be more perfect.

In this sedative and busy life, this book will prove to be a turning point in making you healthy in almost every dimension of your life.

Printed in Great Britain
by Amazon

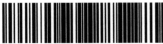